Second Edition

Mosby's

Veterinary PDQ

Veterinary Facts at Hand
Practical · Detailed · Quick

Consultant
Margi Sirois, EdD, MS, RVT

ELSEVIER

3251 Riverport Lane
St. Louis, Missouri 63043

Mosby's Veterinary PDQ   ISBN: 978-0-323-24066-6

Notices

Knowledge and best practice in this field are constantly changing.
As new research and experience broaden our understanding,
changes in research methods, professional practices, or medical
treatment may become necessary.

Practitioners and researchers must always rely on their own
experience and knowledge in evaluating and using any
information, methods, compounds, or experiments described
herein. In using such information or methods they should be
mindful of their own safety and the safety of others, including
parties for whom they have a professional responsibility.

With respect to any drug or pharmaceutical products identified,
readers are advised to check the most current information provided
(i) on procedures featured or (ii) by the manufacturer of each
product to be administered, to verify the recommended dose or
formula, the method and duration of administration, and
contraindications. It is the responsibility of practitioners, relying on
their own experience and knowledge of their patients, to make
diagnoses, to determine dosages and the best treatment for each
individual patient, and to take all appropriate safety precautions.

To the fullest extent of the law, neither the Publisher nor the
authors, contributors, or editors, assume any liability for any injury
and/or damage to persons or property as a matter of products
liability, negligence or otherwise, or from any use or operation of
any methods, products, instructions, or ideas contained in the
material herein.

International Standard Book Number: 978-0-323-24066-6

Vice President and Publisher: Linda Duncan
Content Strategy Director: Penny Rudolph
Content Manager: Shelly Stringer
Publishing Services Manager: Catherine Jackson
Senior Project Manager: David Stein
Design Direction: Amy Buxton

Printed in China
Last digit is the print number: 9 8 7 6 5 4 3

D0102532

Commonly Used Medical Prescription Abbreviations[2]

Abbreviation	Meaning
bid	Twice daily
disp	dispense
g (or gm)	gram
gr	grain
gtt	drop
h (or hr)	hour
IC	intracardiac
IM	intramuscular
IP	intraperitoneal
IV	intravenous
L	liter
mg	milligram
mL (or ml)	milliliter
OD	right eye
OS	left eye
OU	both eyes
PO	by mouth
prn	as needed
q	every
q4h	every 4 hours
qd	every day (daily)
qid	four times daily
qod	every other day
sid	once a day
SQ (or SC)	subcutaneous
stat	immediately
TBL or Tbsp	tablespoon
tid	three times daily
TD	transdermal
TM	transmucosal
tsp	teaspoon

REQUIREMENTS OF PRESCRIPTIONS[2]

- Name of veterinary hospital or veterinarian, address, and telephone number
- Date on which the prescription was written
- Client's (owner's) name and address and species of animal (animal's name optional)
- Rx symbol (from the Latin, meaning *take thou of*)
- Drug name, concentration, and number of units to be dispensed
- Sig (from the Latin *signa*, meaning *write* or *label*), which indicates directions for treatment of the animal
- Signature of the veterinarian
- DEA registration number if the drug is a controlled substance

---

HOMETOWN VETERINARY ASSOCIATES
2000 West Chelsea Ave., Brookside, PA 13233
(324) 555-0214

Date: *November 22, 2001*

Patient: *Cricket*   Species: *Canine*

Owner: *Kathy Gagnier*   Phone: *555-0127*

Address: *2000 Christopher Ln,*
West Brookside, PA 13235

℞ *Amoxicillin tablets 100 mg #30 tabs*
   Sig: 1 tab q8h PO PRN until gone

   <u>*Robert L. Bill*</u> D.V.M.

A hypothetical prescription for a pharmacist.

COMMON MEDICATIONS

Antimicrobials[34A]

Generic Name	Trade Names	Routes	Notes
Aminoglycosides			
Amikacin	Amiglyde-V	IV, IM, SC, intrauterine	Keep animal well hydrated; possible nephrotoxic, ototoxic effects
Gentamicin	Gentocin, Garasol	IV, IM (stings), PO (water additive), topical	Keep animal well hydrated; possible nephrotoxic, ototoxic, neurotoxic effects
Neomycin	Biosol	IV, IM, SC, PO, topical	Not absorbed well systemically; highly nephrotoxic when given parenterally
Penicillins			
Amoxicillin	Amoxi-Tabs, Biomox	IV, IM, SC, PO, intramammary	Give with food if GI upset occurs
Penicillin G	Flocillin, Dual-Pen	IV, IM, SC, PO	Route of administration depends on drug form (potassium, procaine, benzathine)

Penicillins—cont'd			
Amoxicillin with clavulanic acid	Clavamox	PO	An alternative for bacteria that have developed resistance to amoxicillin
Ampicillin	Polyflex	IV (slow), IM, PO	Do not give orally to rabbits
Ampicillin/ sulbactam	Unasyn	IV, IM	Similar activity as clavunalate
Cephalosporins			
Cefadroxil	Cefa-tabs, Cefa-drops	PO	First-generation cephalosporin; cephalosporins should not be used in patients with a known allergy to penicillin
Cefazolin	Ancef, Kefzol	IV (slow), IM, SC	First-generation cephalosporin
Cefovecin sodium	Convenia	SC	Single injection provides 14-day therapeutic level
Cephalexin	Keflex	PO	First-generation cephalosporin
Cefoxitin	Mefoxin	IV, IM, SC	Second-generation cephalosporin

Continued

Antimicrobials[34A]—cont'd

Generic Name	Trade Names	Routes	Notes
Tetracyclines			
Tetracycline	Panmycin	IV (slow), IM, PO	Tetracyclines may cause tooth discoloration in prenatal and neonatal animals
Doxycycline	Vibromycin, Doxirobe gel	IV, PO, periodontal gel	Longer half-life; better central nervous system penetration than tetracycline
Oxytetracycline	Oxytet, Terramycin	IV, IM, PO	Many veterinary products and uses, including feed additive
Quinolones			
Ciprofloxacin	Cipro	IV, IM, SC, PO	Rarely used in veterinary medicine
Enrofloxacin	Baytril, Baytril Otic	IM, PO, topical	Similar to ciprofloxacin; avoid use in patients with renal failure
Orbifloxacin	Orbax	PO	Veterinary drug
Marbofloxacin	Zeniquin	PO	Newest veterinary-approved fluoroquinolone
Moxifloxacin		Ophthalmic	For gram-negative corneal infections

Lincosamides and Macrolides

Clindamycin	Antirobe	IM (stings), SC, PO	Do not administer to rabbits, hamsters, guinea pigs
Azithromycin	Zithromax	PO	Better absorption, longer half-life than erythromycin

Sulfonamides

Sulfadiazine or trimethoprim	Tribrissen, Di-Trim	IV, SC, PO	Can precipitate in the kidneys of dehydrated animals; can cause keratoconjunctivitis sicca
Sulfadimethoxine	Albon	IV, IM, SC, PO	Sulfas are coccidiostatic

Miscellaneous

Metronidazole	Flagyl	IV, PO	Antiprotozoal; may be neurotoxic and immuno-suppressive at higher doses

Antivirals

Idoxuridine, trifluridine		Topical	Ophthalmic antivirals for feline herpes infection
Interferon-α2A	Roferon-A	PO	For treatment of nonneoplastic FELV

Continued

Antimicrobials[34A]—cont'd

Generic Name	Trade Names	Routes	Notes
Antifungals			
Fluconazole	Diflucan	IV, PO	Fungistatic; is probably most useful for central nervous system infections
Griseofulvin	Fulvicin U/F	PO	Known teratogen in cats
Itraconazole	Sporanox	PO	Information on safety and toxicity is limited
Ketaconazole	Nizoral	PO	Less toxic than amphotericin B; used to reduce dosage of cyclosporine
Nystatin	Panalog, Derma-vet, Mycostatin	PO, topical	Used to treat gastrointestinal and skin *Candida* infections
Miconazole	Monistat-1V, Conofite	Topical	Used to treat fungal ophthalmic infections

Antiparasitics for Treating Internal Parasites in Dogs and Cats*

Drug	Toxocara, Toxascaris	Ancylostoma, Uncinaria	Trichuris	Taenia	Dipylidium	Giardia	Coccidia
Albendazole	+	+	+	+	–	+	–
Fenbendazole	+	+	+	+	–	–	–
Furazolidone	–	–	–	–	–	+	+
Ivermectin	+	+	+	–	–	–	–
Metronidazole	–	–	–	–	–	+	–
Milbemycin oxime	+	+	+	–	–	–	–
Praziquantel	–	–	–	+	+	–	–
Selamectin	+	+	–	–	–	–	–
Sulfadiazine or trimethoprim	–	–	–	–	–	–	+
Thiabendazole	–	–	–	–	–	–	–

+, Indicated for use; –, not indicated for use.
*Many of these medications are used in combination with other antiparasitics.

Antiparasitics for Treating External Parasites on Dogs and Cats*[24A]

Drug	Fleas	Lice	Mites	Ticks
Allethrin	+	−	−	−
Amatraz	−	−	+	−
D-Limonene	+	+	−	−
Fipronil	+	+	−	+
Imidacloprid	+	+	−	−
Lime-sulfur	−	−	+	−
Lufenuron	+	−	−	−
Methoprene	+			
Permethrin	+		−	
Pyrethrins	+		−	
Selamectin		−		
Spinosad	+	−	−	−

+, Indicated for use; −, not indicated for use.
*Many of these medications are used in combination with other antiparasitics.

Heartworm Preventives*[2]

Generic Name	Trade Names	Route, Dose Interval	Approved for Use in Dogs	Approved for Use in Cats
Ivermectin	Heartgard and others	By mouth (PO) monthly	Yes	Yes (some products)
Milbemycin oxime	Interceptor and others	PO monthly	Yes	No (doses do exist)
Selamectin	Revolution	Topical monthly	Yes	Yes
Moxidectin	Advantage multi	Topical	Yes	Yes

*Many of these medications are used in combination with other antiparasitics.

Preanesthetics, Sedatives, Anesthetics[34A]

Generic Name	Trade Names	Routes	Notes
Barbiturates			
Pentobarbital	Nembutal	IV (slow to effect)	Used for induction of general anesthesia and to manage status epilepticus; can be used as a single agent for euthanasia; Class II–controlled substance; short-acting agents
Pentobarbital with phenytoin	Beuthanasia-D	IV	For euthanasia only
Thiopental	Pentothal	IV only	May adsorb to plastic IV bags and lines; ultra–short acting
Tranquilizers and Sedatives			
Acepromazine	PromAce, Atravet	IV, IM (stings), SC, PO	Do not use in conjunction with organophosphates; may cause paradoxical central nervous system stimulation, hypotension
Dexmedetomidine	Dexdomitor	IV, IM	Alpha-2 agonist often used as CRI

Diazepam, midazolam	Valium, Versed	IV, IM, PO, rectal	Used as anxiolytic, muscle relaxant, appetite stimulant, perianesthetic, and anticonvulsant
Oxazepam, alprazolam	Serax, Xanax	PO	Used primarily in behavior modification programs
Medetomidine	Domitor	IV, IM	Alpha-2 agonist used for sedation or analgesia in young, healthy animals; adverse effects, such as bradycardia, can be treated by reversing the drug
Xylazine	Rompun, Anased	IV, IM, SC	Alpha-2 agonist used for sedation analgesia in young, healthy animals; available in 20 and 100 mg/ml; check concentration before administering; respiratory depression and vomiting are common side effects and can be treated by reversing the drug

Miscellaneous Anesthetics

| Ketamine | Ketaset, Vetalar | IV, IM | Dissociative anesthetic; most reflexes and muscle tone are maintained; no somatic analgesia exists |

Continued

Preanesthetics, Sedatives, Anesthetics[34A]—cont'd

Generic Name	Trade Names	Routes	Notes
Miscellaneous Anesthetics—cont'd			
Propofol	Rapinovet, PropoFlo, Diprivan	IV only	Rapid induction and recovery; drug is carried in an egglecithin and soy base, which supports bacterial growth
Tiletamine/ zolazepam	Telazol	IV, IM	Tiletamine is a dissociative anesthetic; zolazepam is a tranquilizer; most reflexes are retained
Etomidate	Amidate	IV	Minimal effects on cardiovascular and respiratory system occur; given alone causes myoclonus
Guaifenesin	Guailaxin	IV, PO	Muscle relaxant perianesthetic when given parenterally; expectorant when given orally
Anticonvulsants			
Phenobarbital	Luminal	IV (slow), IM, PO	Is usually the first drug of choice for idiopathic epilepsy; may be used for status seizure; long acting

Anticonvulsants—cont'd

Bromides	Potassium (sodium)	PO	Used as an adjunct in management of idiopathic epilepsy
Clonazepam	Klonopin	PO	Duration of activity may be short in dogs
Diazepam	Valium	IV, rectal, intranasal	Used to control seizures in progress
Pentobarbital	Nembutal	IV	Used in status epilepticus for intractable seizures

Constant Rate Infusions

Dexmedetomidine*	Concentration	CRI Ingredients		Dilution†	Delivery	
	Original 0.50 mg/ml	Dexmedetomidine 500 mcg/ml		500 ml 0.9% NaCl, LRS, NormR	1-3 mcg/kg/hr	
		8 ml	creates 8 mcg/ml		8 mcg/ml	0.1-0.4 ml/kg/hr
		4 ml	creates 4 mcg/ml		4 mcg/ml	0.3-0.8 ml/kg/hr

*Notes: loading dose mcg/kg decreases as body weight increases!
†Remove equal volume fluid prior to adding medications to bag.

Canine or Feline Patient Weight in Kilograms										
	5	10	15	20	25	30	35	40	45	50
Dexmedetomidine 8 mcg/ml CFI in ml/hr	0.5-2.0	1.0-4.0	1.5-6.0	2.0-8.0	2.5-10.0	3.0-12.0	3.5-14.0	4.0-16.0	4.5-18.0	5.0-20.0
Dexmedetomidine 4 mcg/ml CFI in ml/hr	1.5-4.0	3.0-8.0	4.5-12.0	6.0-16.0	7.5-20.0	9.0-24.0	10.5-28.0	12.0-32.0	13.5-36.0	15.0-40.0

http://www.vasg.org/constant_rate_infusions.htm
http://www.cvmbs.colostate.edu/clinsci/wing/fluids/cri.htm
http://www.acvs.org/symposium/proceedings2011/data/papers/157.pdf
Gaynor JS, Muir MW: Handbook of veterinary pain management, St Louis, 2002, Elsevier, pp 152-156, 210-230, 407-410.
Paddleford RR: Manual of small animal anesthesia, ad 2, Philadelphia, 1999, Saunders, pp 19-24.

Constant Rate Infusions—cont'd

Dobutamine	Concentration	Ingredients	Dilution*	Delivery
	Original 12.5 mg/ml	9.6 ml (12.5 mg/ml) dobutamine (total 120 mg)	500 ml 0.9% NaCl, LRS, NormR 0.24 mg/ml 240 mcg/ml	1-10 mcg/kg/min 0.25-2.5 ml/kg/hr 2 mcg/kg/min recommended starting dose (Rosati et al. ACVA Proceedings 2005)

*Remove equal volume fluid prior to adding medications to bag.

Canine or Feline Patient Weight in Kilograms										
	5	10	15	20	25	30	35	40	45	50
Dobutamine CRI in ml/hr	1.25-12.5	2.5-25	3.75-37.5	5-50	6.25-62.5	7.5-75.0	8.75-87.5	10-100	11.5-115	12.75-127.5

http://www.vesc.org/constant_rate_infusions.htm
http://www.cvmbs.colostate.edu/clinsci/wing/fluids/cri.htm
http://www.acvc.org/symposium/proceedings2011/data/papers/157.pdf
Gaynor JS, Muir MW: *Handbook of veterinary pain management*, St Louis, 2002, Elsevier, pp 152-156, 210-230, 4C7-410.
Paddleford RF: *Manual of small animal anesthesia*, ed 2, Philadelphia, 1999, Saunders, pp 19-24.

Constant Rate Infusions—cont'd

Dopamine*	Concentration	Ingredients	Dilution†	Delivery
	Original 40 mg/ml	7.5 ml (40 mg/ml) dopamine (total 300 mg)	500 ml 0.9% NaCl, LRS, NormR	7 mcg/kg/min recommended starting dose (Rosati et al. ACVA Proceedings 2005)
			New concentration: 0.60 mg/ml	2-10 mcg/kg/min
				120-600 mcg/kg/hr
				0.12-0.6 ml/kg/hr
				0.20-1.0 ml/kg/hr

*Notes: dopamine comes in 40, 80, and 160 mg/ml concentrations.
†Remove equal volume fluid prior to adding medications to bag.

Canine or Feline Patient Weight in Kilograms										
	5	10	15	20	25	30	35	40	45	50
Dopamine CRI in ml/hr	1-5	2-10	3-15	4-20	5-25	6-30	7-35	8-40	9-45	10-50

http://www.vasg.org/constant_rate_infusions.htm
http://www.cvmbs.colostate.edu/clinsci/wing/fluids/cri.htm
http://www.acvs.org/symposium/proceedings2011/data/papers/157.pdf
Gaynor JS, Muir MW: *Handbook of veterinary pain management*, St Louis, 2002, Elsevier, pp 152-156, 210-230, 407-410.
Paddleford RR: *Manual of small animal anesthesia*, ed 2, Philadelphia, 1999, Saunders, pp 19-24.

Constant Rate Infusions—cont'd

Fentanyl	Concentration	Loading Dose	CRI*		CRI Delivery Ranges	8 mcg/ml	4 mcg/ml
	0.05 mg/ml	3-5 mcg/kg	Created at 4 mcg/ml or 8 mcg/ml dilution				
			Add either of the following to a 500 ml bag of 0.9% NaCl, NormR, LRS		Analgesia 2-10 mcg/kg/hr	0.25-1.25 ml/kg/hr	0.5-2.5 ml/kg/hr
			80 ml fentanyl	creates 8 mcg/ml			
			40 ml fentanyl	creates 4 mcg/ml	Analgesia 20-40 mcg/kg/hr	2.5-5 ml/kg/hr	5-10 ml/kg/hr
			If a smaller bag or fentanyl volume is necessary, add either of the following to a 250 ml bag of 0.9% NaCl, NormR, LRS				
			40 ml fentanyl	creates 8 mcg/ml			
			20 ml fentanyl	creates 4 mcg/ml			

8 mcg/ml Fentanyl CRI in ml/hr

	Canine or Feline Patient Weight in Kilograms									
	5	10	15	20	25	30	35	40	45	50
Analgesia	1.25-6.25	2.5-12.5	3.75-18.75	5.0-25.0	6.25-31.25	7.5-37.5	8.75-43.75	10-50	11.25-56.25	12.5-62.5
Anesthesia	12.5-25	25-50	37.5-75	50-100	62.5-125	75-150	87.5-175	100-200	125-250	125-500

4 mcg/ml Fentanyl CRI in ml/hr

	Canine or Feline Patient Weight in Kilograms									
	5	10	15	20	25	30	35	40	45	50
Analgesia	2.5-12.5	5-25	7.5-37.5	10-50	12.5-62.5	15-75	17.5-87.5	20-100	22.5-112.5	125-500
Anesthesia	25-50	50-100	75-150	100-200	125-250	150-300	175-350	200-400	225-450	250-500

http://www.vasg.org/constant_rate_infusions.htm

http://www.cvmbs.colostate.edu/clinsci/wing/fluids/cri.htm

http://www.acvs.org/symposium/proceedings2011/data/papers/157.pdf

Gaynor JS, Muir MW: Handbook of veterinary pain management, St Louis, 2002, Elsevier, pp 152-156, 210-230, 197-410.

Paddleford RR: Manual of small animal anesthesia, ec 2, Philadelphia, 1999, Saunders, pp 19-24.

Constant Rate Infusions—cont'd

Fentanyl, Lidocaine, Ketamine (FLK)*	Concentration	Loading Dose	CRI‡		Delivery		Rate
Fentanyl	0.05 mg/ml	3-5 mcg/kg	0.05 mg/ml	30 ml	1.5 mg	0.05-0.15 mcg/kg/min	0.003-0.009 mg/kg/hr	1-3 ml/kg/hr dogs and cats
Lidocaine	20 mg/ml	Dogs 0.5-1.0 mg/kg Cats 0.25 mg/kg	20 mg/ml	12.5 ml	250 mg	8.3-25 mcg/kg/min	0.50-1.5 mg/kg/hr	
Ketamine	100 mg/ml	0.25-0.50 mg/kg	100 mg/ml	1.80 ml	180 mg	2-20 mcg/kg/min	0.12-1.2 mg/kg/hr	

* Notes: light sensitive; in cats, limit high-dose delivery to 2 hours, and subsequent low-dose delivery to an additional 4 hours.
†Created with the following volumes of agents diluted into (total volume) 500 ml of 0.9% NaCl, NormR, LRS.
‡Remove equal volume fluid prior to adding medications to bag.

Canine or Feline Patient Weight in Kilograms									
	5	10	15	20	25	30	35	40	45	50
FLK CRI in ml/hr	5-15	10-30	15-45	20-60	25-75	30-90	35-105	40-120	45-135	50-150

http://www.vesg.org/constant_rate_infusions.htm

http://www.cvmbs.colostate.edu/clinsci/wing/fluids/cri.htm

http://www.acvs.org/symposium/proceedings2011/data/papers/157.pdf

Gaynor JS, Muir MW: Handbook of veterinary pain management, St Louis, 2002, Elsevier, pp 152-156, 210-230 407-410.

Paddleford RR: Manual of small animal anesthesia, ed 2, Philadelphia, 1999, Saunders, pp 19-24.

Constant Rate Infusions—cont'd

Hydromorphone, Lidocaine, Ketamine Combination (HLK)*	Concentration	Loading Dose	CRI‡			Delivery	Rate
Hydromorphone	2 mg/ml hydromorphone	0.5 mg/kg IM or slow IV	15 mg/ml	0.80 ml	12 mg	0.4-1.2 mcg/kg/min	0.024-0.072 mg/kg/hr	Dog or cat 1-3 ml/kg/hr
Lidocaine	20 mg/ml lidocaine	Dogs 0.5-1 mg/kg Cats 0.25 mg/kg	20 mg/ml	12.5 ml	250 mg	8.3-25 mcg/kg/min	0.50-1.5 mg/kg/hr	
Ketamine	100 mg/ml ketamine	0.25 to 0.5 mg/kg	100 mg/ml	1.80 ml	180 mg	2-20 mcg/kg/min	0.12-1.2 mg/kg/hr	

*Notes: in cats, limit high-dose delivery to 2 hours, and subsequent low-dose delivery to an additional 4 hours.
†Created with the following volumes of agents diluted into 500 ml of 0.9% NaCl, NormR, LRS.
‡Remove equal volume fluid prior to adding medications to bag.

Canine or Feline Patient Weight in Kilograms										
	5	10	15	20	25	30	35	40	45	50
HLK CRI in ml/hr	5-15	10-30	15-45	20-60	25-75	30-90	35-105	40-120	45-135	50-150

http://www.vasg.org/constant_rate_infusions.htm
http://www.cvmbs.colostate.edu/clinsci/wing/fluids/cri.htm
http://www.acvs.org/symposium/proceedings2011/data/papers/157.pdf
Gaynor JS, Muir MW: *Handbook of veterinary pain management*, St Louis, 2002, Elsevier, pp 152-156, 210-230 407-410.
Paddleford RR: *Manual of small animal anesthesia*, ed 2, Philadelphia, 1999, Saunders, pp 19-24.

Constant Rate Infusions—cont'd

Methadone*	Concentration	Loading Dose	Ingredients	Dilution†	Delivery
	Original 10 mg/ml	0.1-0.2 mg/kg	8 ml methadone (80 mg)	500 ml 0.9% NaCl, NormR, LRS	0.12-0.2 mg/kg/hr 0.75-1.25 ml/kg/hr

† Remove equal volume fluid prior to adding medications to bag.

Canine or Feline Patient Weight in Kilograms										
	5	10	15	20	25	30	35	40	45	50
Methadone CRI in ml/hr	3.75-6.25	7.5-12.5	11.25-18.75	15-25	18.75-31.25	22.5-37.5	26.25-43.75	30-50	33.75-56.25	37.5-62.5

http://www.vasg.org/constant_rate_infusions.htm
http://www.cvmbs.colostate.edu/clinsci/wing/fluids/cri.htm
http://www.acvs.org/symposium/proceedings2011/data/papers/157.pdf
Gaynor JS, Muir MW: Handbook of veterinary pain management, St Louis, 2002, Elsevier, pp 152-156, 210-230, 407-410.
Paddleford RR: Manual of small animal anesthesia, ed 2, Philadelphia, 1999, Saunders, pp 19-24.

Constant Rate Infusions—cont'd

Metoclopramide*	Concentration	Ingredients	Dilution†	Delivery
	Original 5 mg/ml	4 ml metoclopramide (20 mg)	500 ml 0.9% NaCl, NormR, LRS	1-2 mg/kg/day
				0.04-0.08 mg/kg/hr
				1-2 ml/kg/hr

*Notes: Light sensitive.
†Remove 4 ml from bag before adding medications.

Canine or Feline Patient Weight in Kilograms										
	5	10	15	20	25	30	35	40	45	50
Metoclopramide CRI in ml/hr	5-10	10-20	15-30	20-40	25-50	30-60	35-70	40-80	45-90	50-100

http://www.vasg.org/constant_rate_infusions.htm
http://www.cvmls.colostate.edu/clinsci/wing/fluids/cri.htm
http://www.acvs.org/symposium/proceedings2011/data/papers/157.pdf
Gaynor JS, Muir WW: *Handbook of veterinary pain management*, St Louis, 2002, Elsevier, pp 152-156, 210-230, 407-410.
Paddleford RR: *Manual of small animal anesthesia*, ed 2, Philadelphia, 1999, Saunders, pp 19-24.

Constant Rate Infusions—cont'd

Morphine, Lidocaine, Ketamine Combination (MLK)*	Concentration	Loading Dose	CRI‡			Delivery	Rate
Morphine	15 mg/ml morphine	0.5 mg/kg IM or slow IV	15 mg/ml	4 ml	60 mg	2-6 mcg/kg/min	Dogs or cats 1-3 ml/kg/hr
Lidocaine	20 mg/ml lidocaine	Dogs 0.5-1 mg/kg Cats 0.25 mg/kg	20 mg/ml	12.5 ml	250 mg	8.3-25 mcg/kg/min	
Ketamine	100 mg/ml ketamine	0.25 to 0.5 mg/kg	100 mg/ml	1.80 ml	180 mg	2-20 mcg/kg/min	

*Notes: in cats, limit high-dose delivery to 2 hours, and subsequent low-dose delivery to an additional 4 hours.
†Created with the following volumes of agents diluted into 500 ml of 0.9% NaCl, NormR, LRS.
‡Remove equal volume fluid prior to adding medications to bag.

Canine or Feline Patient Weight in Kilograms									
	5	10	15	20	25	30	35	40	45	50
MLK CRI in m /hr	5-15	10-30	15-45	20-60	25-75	30-90	35-105	40-120	45-135	50-150

http://www.vasg.org/constant_rate_infusions.htm

http://www.cvmbs.colostate.edu/clinsci/wing/fluids/cri.htm

http://www.acvs.org/symposium/proceedings2011/data/papers/157.pdf

Gaynor JS, Muir MW: *Handbook of veterinary pain management*, St Louis, 2002, Elsevier, pp 152-156, 210-230, 407-410.

Paddleford RR: *Manual of small animal anesthesia*, ed 2, Philadelphia, 1999, Saunders, pp 19-24.

Constant Rate Infusions—cont'd

Propofol*	Concentration	Loading Dose†	CRI	
	10 mg/ml injection (PropoFlo, PropoFlo 28, Rapinovet)	4-6 mg/kg IV slow	Created with nondiluted propofol for IV delivery ranges	
			Sedation	0.1-0.3 mg/kg/min
			Anesthesia	0.4-0.6 mg/kg/min

*Notes: Sedation dose can be helpful as adjunct agent for difficult anesthetic cases or for tracheostomy cases.
Anesthesia dose can be used as TIVA for MRI, vent cases, refractory seizures, or surgery (with addition of analgesia).
Avoid repeated dosing in felines (may contribute to Heinz body anemia).
†For anesthetic induction; if patient is already anesthetized, this may not be necessary.

Propofol CRI in ml/hr	Canine or Feline Patient Weight in Kilograms									
	5	10	15	20	25	30	35	40	45	50
Sedation	3-9	6-18	9-27	12-24	15-36	18-54	21-63	24-72	27-81	30-90
Anesthesia	12-18	24-36	36-54	48-72	60-90	72-108	84-126	96-144	108-162	120-180

Propofol CRI in ml/min	Canine or Feline Patient Weight in Kilograms									
	5	10	15	20	25	30	35	40	45	50
Sedation	0.05-0.15	0.10-0.3	0.15-0.45	0.2-0.6	0.25-0.60	0.30-0.9	0.35-1.05	0.40-1.20	0.45-1.35	0.50-1.50
Anesthesia	0.2-0.3	0.4-0.6	0.6-0.9	0.3-1.2	1.0-1.5	1.2-1.8	1.4-2.10	1.6-2.40	1.8-2.70	2.0-3.0

http://www.vasg.org/constant_rate_infusions.htm

http://www.cvmbs.colostate.edu/clinsci/wing/fluids/cri.htm

http://www.acvs.org/symposium/proceedings2011/data/papers/157.pdf

Gaynor JS, Muir MW: Handbook of veterinary pain management, St Louis, 2002, Elsevier, pp 152-156, 210-230, 407-410.

Paddleford RR: Manual of small animal anesthesia, ed 2, Philadelphia, 1999, Saunders, pp 19-24.

Inhalant Anesthetics[25A]

Isoflurane	Sevoflurane
Muscle Relaxation	
Good	Moderate
Effect on Nondepolarizing Muscle Relaxants	
Greatly increased	Probably increased
Analgesia	
Slight	Slight
Effect on Respiration	
Depression	Depression
Effect on Heart	
Slight	Slight
Potential for Causing Cardiac Arrhythmias	
None reported	Sensitizes myocardium to catecholamine-induced arrhythmias
Effect on Blood Pressure	
Decreases	Decreases
Elimination from the Body	
Respiration 99%	Respiration 97%
Lipid Solubility	
Low	Low
Maintenance Range	
1.5%-2.5%	2.5%-4.0%

Analgesic and Antiinflammatory Agents[34A]

Nonsteroidal Antiinflammatory Drugs (NSAIDs)

Generic Name	Trade Names	Routes	Notes
Acetylsalicylic acid	Aspirin	PO	Analgesic, antiinflammatory, and antipyretic; can use with caution in cats; enteric coating prevents gastric irritation
Carprofen	Rimadyl	IV, IM, SC, PO	Labrador retriever may be more prone to severe side effects
Deracoxib	Deramaxx	PO	COX-1 sparing; approved for dogs only
Etodolac	EtoGesic, Lodine	PO	COX-2 selective; approved for dogs only
Firocoxib	Previcox	PO	COX-2 selective; chewable tablets; approved for dogs only
Ketoprofen	Ketofen, Orudis	IV, IM, SC, PO	
Meloxicam	Metacam	IV, SC, PO, TM	COX-2 selective; used for chronic or acute musculoskeletal disorders; approved for use in cats

Continued

Analgesic and Antiinflammatory Agents[34A]—cont'd

Generic Name	Trade Names	Routes	Notes
Nonsteroidal Antiinflammatory Drugs (NSAIDs)—cont'd			
Piroxicam	Feldene	PO	Use in cats is as an antineoplastic agent
Tepoxalin	Zubrin	PO	COX and LOX inhibitor; rapidly disintegrating tablets for dogs
Tolfenamic acid	Tolfedine	IM, SC, PO	Pharmacologically similar to aspirin; approved for dogs and cats in Canada and Europe
Tramadol	Ultram	PO	Used for management of chronic and acute pain
Dimethyl sulfoxide (DMSO)		IV, topical	Teratogenic in some species; wear gloves when applying
Corticosteroids			
Dexamethasone	Azium, Dexasone	IV, IM, SC, PO	Long acting
Methylprednisolone	Medrol, Depo-Medrol, Solu-Medrol	IM, SC, PO	Intermediate acting

Prednisolore sodium succinate	Solu-Delta-Cortef	IV, IM	Intermediate acting
Triamcinolone	Vetalog	IM, SC, PO	Intermediate acting
Prednisone	Meticorten, Deltasone	IV, IM, SC, PO	Intermediate acting
Hydrocortisone	Cortef	IV, IM, PO	Short acting
Glycosaminoglycans			
Glucosamine	Many	PO	Often combined with chondroitin, these agents are considered nutraceuticals, not drugs
PSGAG	Adequan	IM	Postinjection inflammation is possible when administered into the joint
Pentosan polysulfate	Cartrophen-Vet (outside U.S.), Elmiron	IM, SC, PO	Used for osteoarthritis and interstitial cystitis (cats)

Continued

Analgesic and Antiinflammatory Agents[34A]—cont'd

Generic Name	Trade Names	Routes	Notes
Muscle Relaxants, Opioid (Narcotic) Analgesics			
Methocarbamol	Robaxin-V	IV, PO	Skeletal muscle relaxant, may cause sedation
Butorphanol	Torbutrol, Torbugesic, Dolorex	IV, IM, SC, PO	Partial agonist or antagonist; poorly absorbed from gastrointestinal tract; also used as an antitussive
Buprenorphine	Buprenex	IV, IM, SC, TM	Partial agonist; may cause respiratory depression; TM administration is unreliable in dogs
Fentanyl	Duragesic	Transdermal; also IV, epidural	Continuous, sustained analgesia

Hydromorphone	Dilaudid	IV, IM, SC, rectal	μ agonist; may cause panting, then respiratory depression; Class II controlled substance
Methadone	Dolophine	IV, IM, SC	Synthetic opioid; less likely to induce vomiting than other opioids
Morphine	Infumorph	IM, IV	Vomiting usually occurs
	Duramorph	Epidural	Preservative-free; extra-label use

Parenteral Fluids[1]

Fluid	Content	Tonicity	pH	Osmolality
Lactated Ringer's solution	Na^+, K^+, CA^{++}, Cl^-, lactate	Isotonic	6.7	273
Plasmalyte A	Na^+, K^+, Cl^-, Mg^{++}, glucose	Isotonic	7.4	294
Sodium chloride 0.45%	Na^+, Cl^-	Hypotonic	5.0	155
Sodium chloride 0.9%	Na^+, Cl^-	Isotonic	5.0	310
Dextrose 5%	Glucose	Hypotonic	5.0	253
Dextrose 2.5% with 0.45% sodium chloride	Na^+, Cl^-, glucose	Isotonic	4.5	280

Blood Products[1]

Contents	Shelf Life	Preparation	Comments
Fresh Whole Blood (FWB)			
RBCs, plasma proteins, coagulation factors, WBCs, platelets	Less than 8 hours after initial collection	Use immediately after collection	Restores blood volume and oxygen-carrying capacity
Stored Whole Blood (WB)			
RBC, plasma proteins	Up to 42 days (dependent on anticoagulant and preservative used); refrigerate at 1°-6° C	Bring to room temperature before using	Restores blood volume and O₂-carrying capacity, WBC and platelets not viable; factors V and VII diminished
Packed Red Blood Cells (PRBC)			
RBC	Dependent on anticoagulant used; refrigerate at 1°-6° C	Bring to room temperature before using	Same O₂-carrying capacity as WB but with less volume

Continued

Blood Products[1]—cont'd

Contents	Shelf Life	Preparation	Comments
PRBC, Adenine-Saline Added			
RBC, reduced plasma, 100 ml additive solution	28-30 days; refrigerate at 1°-6° C	Bring to room temperature before using	Additive solution extends shelf life; reduces viscosity for infusion
Platelet-Rich Plasma (PRP)/Platelet Concentrate			
Platelets, few RBCs and WBCs, some plasma	5 days at 22° C; intermittent agitation required	Administer immediately after collection and preparation	Should not refrigerate
Fresh Frozen Plasma (FFP)			
Plasma, albumin, coagulation factors	12 months frozen at −18° C or colder	Thaw in 37° C warm-water bath	Frozen within 8 hours after collection; no platelets; administer within 4 hours of thawing

FP

Plasma, albumin, stable coagulation factors	5 years frozen at −18° C or colder	Thaw in 37° C warm-water bath	Frozen after more than 8 hours after collection; no platelets; administer within 4 hours of thawing

Cryoprecipitate (Cryo)

Factor VIII, von Willebrand's factor, fibrinogen, fibronectin	12 months frozen at −18° C or colder	Thaw in 37° C warm-water bath	Administer within 4 hours of thawing

Cardiovascular Drugs[34]

Generic Name	Trade Names	Routes	Notes
Inotropic			
Digoxin	Lanoxin, Cardoxin	IV, PO	Toxic and therapeutic doses may overlap Dobermans tend to be sensitive to digoxin
Dobutamine	Dobutrex	IV infusion	Use diluted solutions within 24 hours
Pimobendan	Vetmedin	PO	Used to manage congestive heart failure; available in Canada and Europe
Adrenergics			
Epinephrine	Adrenalin	IV, IM, SC IT IC Inhalation	Available in several sizes for various uses: 1:100 (1% or 10 mg/ml) topical, inhalation 1:1000 (0.1% or 1 mg/ml) IV, IM, SC, IT 1:10,000 (0.01% or 0.1 mg/ml) IV, IC
Dopamine	Intropin	IV infusion	Effects are dose dependent
Anticholinergics			
Atropine	Many	IV, IM, SC	Used for cardiac support

Glycopyrrolate	Robinul-V	IV, IM, SC	Used for cardiac support; not suitable for emergency use
β-Blockers			
Atenolol	Tenormin	Oral	Can disrupt blood sugar control in diabetic patients
Propranolol	Inderal	IV (slow), PO	Can be blocked by β-blocker antiarrhythmics
Metoprolol	Lopressor, Toprol	PO	Similar to propranolol, safer for patients with bronchoconstriction
Sotalol	Betapace, Cardol	PO	Similar to propranolol
Calcium Channel Blockers			
Amlodipine	Norvasc	PO	Use cautiously in animals with heart failure
Diltiazem	Cardizem	PO	Toxicity may be treated with calcium infusion
Angiotensin-Converting Enzyme (ACE)			
Benazapril	Lotensin	PO	For adjunctive treatment of heart failure

Continued

Cardiovascular Drugs[34]—cont'd

Generic Name	Trade Names	Routes	Notes
ACE Inhibitors			
Enalapril	Enacard, Vasotec	IV, PO	Give on an empty stomach
Vasodilators			
Hydralazine	Apresolene	IM, PO	Use cautiously in patients with severe renal disease
Nitroglycerin	Nitro-Bid, Nitrol	Topical	Wear gloves when applying ointment
Antiarrhythmics			
Lidocaine	Xylocaine	IV	Do not use lidocaine with epinephrine preparations for intravenous solutions
Procainamide	Pronestyl, Procan	IV, IM, PO	Use with caution with other antiarrhythmics
Quinidine	Quinidex	IV, IM, PO	Use with caution with other antiarrhythmics

Diuretics

Furosemide	Lasix, Disal, Diuride, Salix	IV, IM, PO	Veterinary preparations are normally slightly yellow; if human preparations turn yellow, do not use
Spironolactone	Aldactone	PO	Potassium-sparing diuretic
Mannitol	Osmitrol, Mannitrol	IV infusion	Primary use is to decrease intracranial pressure

Anticoagulants

Heparin	Many	SC	Used in DIC and in IV flush solutions
Dalteparin, Enoxaparin	Fragmin, Lovenox	SC	LMWH used to prevent thromboembolisms

Respiratory Drugs[34]

Generic Name	Trade Names	Routes	Notes
Bronchodilators			
Albuterol	Ventolin, Proventil	PO, inhalation	Most adverse effects are dose related and generally transient
Terbutaline	Brethine	SC, PO, inhalation	
Metaproterenol	Alupent	PO, inhalation	
Aminophylline	Many	IV, IM (painful), PO	Do not inject air into multidose vials; CO_2 causes drug to precipitate; narrow therapeutic index
Theophylline		IV, IM, PO	Available in sustained-release oral dose form
Inhaled Steroids			
Fluticasone	Flovent	MDI	Use a spacer for administration
Beclomethasone	Vanceril, QVAR	MDI	Use a spacer for administration

Antihistamines

Chlorpheniramine	Many	PO	Do not allow time-released capsules to dissolve before oral administration
Cyproheptadine	Periactin	PO	Also used for appetite stimulation in cats
Diphenhydramine	Benadryl	IV, IM, PO	IV form used to counteract anaphylactic reactions
Hydroxyzine	Atarax	PO	All antihistamines may cause sedation
Clemastine	Tavist	PO	Do not use the over-the-counter product Tavist-D
Trimeprazine (with prednisolone)	Temaril-P	PO	Combination antihistamine and corticosteroid

Antitussives

Butorphanol	Torbutrol, Torbugesic	IV, IM, SC, PO	Narcotic cough suppressant
Codeine	Many	PO	Cough syrups containing codeine are usually combination drug products
Hydrocodone	Hycodan, Tussigon	PO	Narcotic cough suppressant

Continued

Respiratory Drugs[34]—cont'd

Generic Name	Trade Names	Routes	Notes
Antitussives—cont'd			
Dextromethorphan	Robitussin	PO	Nonnarcotic cough suppressant; available over the counter
Decongestants			
Phenylpropanola-mine	Propagest, Proin	PO	Most common use in veterinary medicine is to treat urinary incontinence
Mucolytics			
Acetylcysteine	Mucomyst	IV, PO, inhalation	Antidote for acetaminophen toxicity
Stimulants			
Doxapram	Dopram	IV, SC, sublingual	Use in newborn resuscitation is controversial

Gastrointestinal Drugs[34]

Generic Name	Trade Names	Routes	Notes
Antiemetics			
Maropitant citrate	Cerenia	SC, PO	Prevent and treat acute vomiting; treat motion sickness
Chlorpromazine	Thorazine	IV, IM, PO, rectal	Protect from light; may discolor urine to a pink or red-brown
Dimenhydrinate	Dramamine	PO	Used primarily for motion sickness
Dolasetron	Anzemet	IV, IM, SC	Similar to ondansetron with once-daily dosing
Meclizine	Antivert	PO	Primarily used for motion sickness
Metoclopramide	Reglan	IV (slow), IM, SC, PO	Promotility agent; inhibits gastroesophageal reflux
Ondansetron	Zofran	IV, PO	Indicated for refractory vomiting, chemotherapy sickness, and other hard-to-treat nausea
Prochlorperazine	Compazine	IM, SC, PO, rectal	Rectal suppositories available for at home use in vomiting animals

Continued

Gastrointestinal Drugs[34]—cont'd

Generic Name	Trade Names	Routes	Notes
Antiulcer			
Antacids	Amphogel, Maalox, Basalgel, Tums	PO	Neutralize acid; can affect absorption rates of other oral medications
Cimetidine	Tagamet	IV, IM (stings), SC, PO	Oral form available over the counter; do not refrigerate injectable form
Famotidine	Pepcid	IV, IM, SC, PO	Oral form available over the counter
Nizatidine	Axid	PO	Similar to ranitidine with prokinetic activity
Ranitidine	Zantac	IV (slow), IM (stings), SC, PO	Reduces gastric acid output
Sucralfate	Carafate	PO	Forms a protective barrier at gastric ulcer site; administer 60 minutes before other medications or food

Misoprostol	Cytotec	PO	May cause gastrointestinal side effects such as diarrhea
Omeprazole	Prilosec	PO	A proton-pump inhibitor, may affect absorption rates of drugs requiring a low stomach pH; do not split caplets
Appetite Stimulants			
Cyproheptadine	Periactin	PO	Appetite stimulation in cats; may take more than one dose to be effective
Diazepam	Valium	IV	Appetite stimulation in cats effective immediately after injection; dose is a fraction of that used for sedation
Oxazepam	Serax	PO	Appetite stimulation in cats
Antispasmodics			
Aminopentamide	Centrine	IM, SC, PO	Hypomotility drug; discontinue if urine retention is noted as a side effect

Continued

Gastrointestinal Drugs[34]—cont'd

Generic Name	Trade Names	Routes	Notes
Stimulants			
Metoclopramide	Reglan	IV (slow), IM, SC, PO	Do not use if gastrointestinal obstruction is suspected
Cisapride		PO	Has been removed from U.S. market; used in management of feline chronic constipation
Laxatives			
Magnesium salts	Milk of Magnesia	PO	Hyperosmotic; holds water in gastrointestinal tract and softens stool
Bisacodyl	Dulcolax	PO, rectal suppository	Stimulant laxative
Lactulose	Enulose	PO	Hyperosmotic; also used to reduce blood ammonia levels in hepatic disease
Docusate	Colace, DSS	PO, enema	Stool softener; watch hydration status

Antidiarrheals			
Diphenoxylate/ atropine	Lomotil	PO	Opiates reduce gut motility; small amount of atropine reduces other narcotic effects
Kaolin/pectin	Kaopectate, K-P-Sol	PO	
Bismuth subsalicylate	Pepto-Bismol	PO	May discolor the stool to black
Emetics			
Apomorphine		IV, IM, SC, topically in conjunctiva	If vomiting does not occur with initial dose, subsequent doses are not likely to be effective and may induce toxicity; wear gloves when handling
Miscellaneous			
Ursodiol	Actigall	PO	Use to increase the flow of bile
SAMe	Denosyl	PO	Nutraceutical agent used as an adjunct to treatment of liver disease

Continued

Gastrointestinal Drugs[34]—cont'd

Generic Name	Trade Names	Routes	Notes
Miscellaneous—cont'd			
Pancreatic pancrezyme	Viokase	PO	Products contain lipase, amylase, protease enzymes; cats strongly dislike the taste of powder forms
Activated charcoal	Toxiban, Liquichar	PO	Adsorbant used to prevent absorption of toxic elements in the gastrointestinal tract

Endocrine Drugs[34]

Generic Name	Trade Names	Routes	Notes
Estrogens			
Estradiol	ECP	IM	Primarily used to induce estrus; prevents pregnancy after mismating in dog and cat (rare use); toxic to bone marrow; contraindicated in pregnancy

Diethylstilbestrol (DES)		PO	Used to treat estrogen-responsive urinary incontinence and other conditions in dogs and cats; toxic to bone marrow; contraindicated in pregnancy; banned in food animals
Progestins			
Megestrol	Ovaban, Megace	PO	For false pregnancy, control of estrus cycle; contraindicated in pregnancy; can induce hypo-adrenocorticism, personality changes, transient diabetes, and has many other side effects
Medroxy-progesterone	Depo-Provera	IM, SC, PO	Used in treatment of some behavioral and dematologic conditions; many sice effects
Pituitary Hormones			
Desmopress n	DDAVP	SC, intranasal	Antidiuretic hormone used in the control of diabetes insipidus
Oxytocin	Pitocin	IV, IM, SC	Induction and enhancement of uterine contractions at parturition

Continued

Endocrine Drugs[34]—cont'd			
Generic Name	Trade Names	Routes	Notes
Pituitary Hormones—cont'd			
Corticotropin	Cortrosyn	IV, IM	Used in the ACTH stimulation test
Steroids			
Fludrocortisone	Florinef	PO	Mineralocorticoid for the treatment of hypoadreno-corticism
Desoxycortico-sterone (DOCP)	Percorten-V	IM	Mineralocorticoid for the treatment of hypoadreno-corticism
Stanozolol	Winstrol	PO	Anabolic steroid; rarely used; U.S. controlled drug
Steroid Inhibitors			
Mitotane, Trilostane	Lysodren, Vetoryl	PO	For treatment of pituitary-dependent hyperadreno-corticism; trilostane must be imported in the United States

Seleginine (l-deprenyl)	Anipryl, Eldepryl	PO	For the treatment of hyperadrenocorticism; also used in the treatment of canine cognitive dysfunction
Antidiabetics			
Insulin	Many	SC	Store in refrigerator; mix gently—do not shake before using; clients should be given thorough instructions on the use of insulin
Glipizide, Glyburide	Glucotrol, Micronase	PO	Oral hypoglycemic agents
Drugs Affecting the Thyroid			
Levothyroxine	Soloxine, Thyrozine	PO	T_4 thyroid hormone supplement
Liothyronine	Cytobin	PO	T_3 hormone supplement; may be useful in hypo-thyroid cases that do not respond to T_4
Methimazole	Tapazole	PO	Used in the medical management of hyperthyroidism

Antidotes and Reversing Agents[25A]

Generic Name	Trade Names	Uses and Indications
Acetylcysteine	Mucomyst	Acetaminophen toxicity
Atipamezole	Antisedan	Reversal of medetomidine (Domitor)
Atropine	Many	Organophosphate toxicity
Calcium EDTA	Calcium Disodium Versenate	Lead poisoning
Fomepizole (4-MP)	Antizol-Vet	Ethylene glycol toxicity
Methylene blue	Urolene Blue	Reversal of benzodiazepines (Valium)
Naloxone	Narcan	Ethylene glycol toxicity
Yohimbine	Yobine	Reversal of xylazine (Rompun)

MEDICAL MATH

Conversion Factors[2]

Weight or Mass

1 kilogram (kg) = 2.2 pounds (lb)	
1 kilogram (kg) = 1000 grams (g)	
1 kilogram (kg) = 1,000,000 milligrams (mg)	
1 gram (g) = 1000 milligrams (mg)	
1 gram (g) = 0.001 kilogram (kg)	
1 milligram (mg) = 0.001 gram (g)	
1 milligram (mg) = 1000 micrograms (μg or mcg)	
1 pound (lb) = 0.454 kilogram (kg)	
1 pound (lb) = 16 ounces (oz)	
1 grain (gr) = 64.8 milligrams (mg) (household system)	
1 grain (gr) = 60 milligrams (mg) (apothecary)	

Volume

1 liter (L) = 1000 milliliters (ml)	
1 liter (L) = 10 deciliters (dl)	
1 milliliter (ml) = 1 cubic centimeter (cc)	
1 milliliter (ml) = 1000 microliters (μl or mcl)	
1 tablespoon (TBL or Tbsp) = 3 teaspoons (tsp)	
1 tablespoon (TBL or Tbsp) = 15 milliliters (ml)	
1 teaspoon (tsp) = 5 milliliters (ml)	
1 gallon (gal) = 3.786 liters (L)	
1 gallon (gal) = 4 quarts (qt)	
1 gallon (gal) = 8 pints (pt)	
1 pint (pt) = 2 cups (c)	
1 pint (pt) = 16 fluid ounces (fl oz)	
1 pint (pt) = 473 milliliters (ml)	

Dosage Calculations[2]

$$\text{Dose (Mass)} \times \frac{\text{Volume}}{\text{Mass of Drug}} = \begin{array}{l}\text{Amount} \\ \text{of dose form} \\ \text{to be given}\end{array}$$

$$\text{Dose (Mass)} \times \frac{\text{Tablet}}{\text{Mass of Drug}} = \begin{array}{l}\text{Amount} \\ \text{of dose form} \\ \text{to be given}\end{array}$$

$$\frac{\text{\# Tablet}}{\text{Dose}} \times \frac{\text{\# Doses}}{\text{Day}} = \begin{array}{l}\text{Total tablets} \\ \text{dispensed}\end{array}$$

Fluid Therapy Calculations[23]

Calculations of Fluid Requirements

Body weight (kg) × % dehydration =
ml fluid deficit*

(60 to 80 ml/kg) × Body weight (kg) =
ml of daily fluid requirement*

Free-Drip Calculations

$$\text{Drops per minute} = \frac{\text{Total infusion volume} \times \text{drops/ml}}{\text{Total infusion time (min)}}$$

*Estimation of ongoing losses × 2 = ml of ongoing losses.

Intravenous Fluid Rate Calculations[1A]

ml/hr	60 DROPS/ml	
	drops/min	sec-drop
5	5	12
10	10	6
15	15	4
20	20	3
25	25	2
30	30	2
35	35	2
40	40	2
45	45	1.5
50	50	1
55	55	1
60	60	—

Nutritional Calculations[34]

Resting Energy Requirements (RER)

$70 \times$ Weight $(kg)^{0.75}$ or $30 \times$ (Weight in kg) $+ 70$

Maintenance Energy Requirements (MER)

Canine Feeding Guide

Puppies	<4 months of age $3 \times$ RER >4 months of age $2 \times$ RER
Adult	$1.6 \times$ RER
Senior	$1.4 \times$ RER
Weight prevention	$1.4 \times$ RER
Weight loss	$1.0 \times$ RER
Gestation (last 21 days)	$3.0 \times$ RER
Lactation	4.0 to $8.0 \times$ RER

Feline Feeding Guide

Kittens	$2.5 \times$ RER
Adult	$1.2 \times$ RER
Weight prevention	$1.0 \times$ RER
Weight loss	$0.8 \times$ RER
Breeding	$1.6 \times$ RER
Gestation (gradual increase)	$2.0 \times$ RER
Lactation	2.0 to $6.0 \times$ RER

Animal Care

ANATOMICAL PLANES OF REFERENCE[5,21]

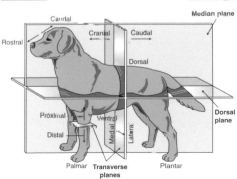

PHYSICAL EXAMINATION PROCEDURES[29]

- Record temperature, pulse, and respiration (TPR)
- Record general condition (e.g., disposition, activity level, overall body condition)
- Evaluate and record condition of each body system:
  - **Integument:** Hydration status, condition of hair coat, alopecia, parasites, lumps, wounds, and rashes
  - **Respiratory:** Respiratory rate and rhythm; rales, ronchi, crepitus, dyspnea, and nasal discharge
  - **Cardiovascular:** Cardiac rate and rhythm; capillary refill time (CRT) and pulse (e.g., rate, character)
  - **Gastrointestinal:** Diarrhea, vomiting abdominal tenderness, and impaction
  - **Genitourinary:** Males—presence or absence of testicles in scrotum, penile discharge. Females—evidence of pregnancy, lactation, vaginal discharge
  - **Musculoskeletal:** Presence or absence of swelling; gait, limping, guarding, tenderness; and overall musculature
  - **Nervous:** Presence or absence of head tilt, tremors; evaluation of pupillary light reflexes and triceps, patellar, and gastrocnemius reflexes
  - **Eyes:** Presence or absence of abrasions, ulcers, discharge
  - **Ears:** Presence or absence of tenderness, parasites, odor, ulcers, discharge
  - **Mucosa:** Color of mucous membranes, odor of mouth, periodontal tissues
  - **Lymphatic:** Size and location of peripheral lymph nodes

Assessment of Level of Consciousness (LOC)[33]

Signs	LOC (Traditional)	AVPU Scale
Fully conscious, alert, engaged and interested in the environment.	Bright, alert, responsive (B/A/R)	A (Alert)
Fully conscious and alert but not engaged, owing to fear, pain, illness, or any other cause. Subdued or quiet.	Quiet, alert, responsive (Q/A/R)	A (Alert)
Mildly depressed. Is aware of surroundings. Can be aroused with minimal difficulty (verbal or tactile stimulus).	Lethargic	A (Alert)
Very depressed. Uninterested in surroundings. Responds to but cannot be fully aroused by a verbal or tactile stimulus.	Obtunded	V (Responds to a verbal stimulus)
A sleeplike state. Nonresponsive to a verbal stimulus. Can be aroused only by a painful stimulus.	Stuporous	P (Responds only to a painful stimulus)
Sleeplike state. Cannot be aroused by any means.	Comatose	U (Unresponsive)

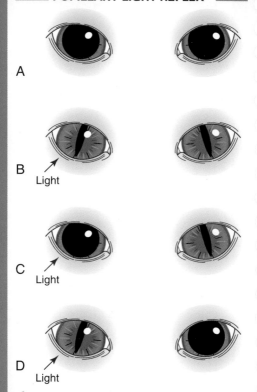

A, Normal pupils. **B**, Direct and consensual light reflex (normal). **C**, Consensual but no direct light reflex (abnormal). **D**, Direct but no consensual light reflex (abnormal).

LOCATION

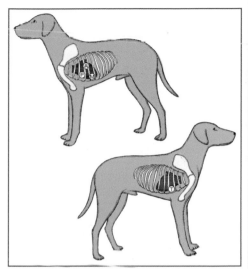

Location of heart valves as an aid in the determination of the origin of a heart murmur. *A*, Aortic; *M*, mitral; *P*, pulmonic; *T*, tricuspid.

The valve area over which the murmur is loudest is usually:
- Aortic
- Mitral
- Tricuspid
- Pulmonic

The location may also be described in relation to chest structures, such as the sternal border.

TIMING

Timing refers to the part of the cardiac cycle during which the murmur is heard:

- Systole
- Diastole
- Continuous

DURATION

Duration refers to the interval within systole or diastole in which the murmur is heard:

- Early systole
- Holosystolic (pansystolic)
- Diastole

CHARACTER

Character refers to the quality of the murmur:

- Plateau or regurgitant type (same sound for the duration of the murmur)
- Decrescendo, crescendo, crescendo-decrescendo, or ejection type (intensity changes throughout the duration of the murmur)
- Machinery (heard throughout systole and diastole)
- Decrescendo or blowing

GRADE

1/6—Can be heard in a quiet room only after several minutes of listening.

2/6—Can be heard immediately but is very soft.

3/6—Has low-to-moderate intensity.

4/6—Is loud but does not have a palpable thrill.

5/6—Is loud with a palpable thrill.

6/6—Can be heard with the stethoscope bell slightly off the thoracic wall.

Estimating Degree of Dehydration[29]

Degree of Dehydration	Clinical Signs
<5%	Not clinically detectable
5% to 6%	Subtle loss of skin elasticity
6% to 8%	Obvious delay in return of tented skin to normal position Slightly prolonged capillary refill time Eyes possibly sunken in orbits Possibly dry mucous membranes
10% to 12%	Skin remains tented Very prolonged capillary refill time Eyes sunken in orbits Dry mucous membranes Possible signs of shock (tachycardia; cool extremities; rapid, weak pulse)
12% to 15%	Obvious signs of shock Death imminent

BODY CONDITION SCORING SYSTEM[39]

Body Condition Scores (Canine)

BCS 1
Thin

- Ribs, lumbar vertebrae, and pelvic bones visible at a distance and felt without pressure
- No palpable fat over tail base, spine, or ribs
- Diminished muscle mass
- Extreme concave abdominal tuck when viewed from side
- Severe hourglass shape when viewed from above

BCS 2
Underweight

- Ribs palpable with little pressure; may be visible
- Minimal palpable fat over ribs, spine, tail base
- Increased concave abdominal tuck when viewed from side
- Marked hourglass shape when viewed from above

BCS 3
IDEAL

- Ribs and spine palpable with slight pressure but not visible; no excess fat covering
- Ribs can be seen with motion of dog
- Good muscle tone apparent
- Concave abdominal tuck when viewed from side
- Hourglass shape to waist when viewed from above

**BCS 4
Overweight**

- Ribs palpable with increased pressure; not visible and have excess fat covering
- Ribs not seen with motion of the dog
- General hefty appearance
- Abdominal concave tuck is reduced or absent when viewed from the side
- Loss of hourglass shape to waist with back slightly broadened when viewed from above

**BCS 5
Obese**

- Ribs and spine not palpable under a heavy fat covering
- Fat deposits visible over lumbar area, tail base, and spine
- Loss of fourglass shape to waist
- Complete loss of abdominal tuck with rounded abdomen
- Back is markedly broadened

Body Condition Scores (Feline)

BCS 1 — Thin

- Ribs, lumbar vertebrae, and pelvic bones visible at a distance and felt without pressure
- No palpable fat over tail base, spine, or ribs
- Diminished muscle mass
- Extreme concave abdominal tuck when viewed from side
- Extreme hourglass shape when viewed from above

BCS 2 — Underweight

- Ribs palpable with little pressure; may be visible
- Minimal palpable fat over ribs, spine, tail base
- Increased concave abdominal tuck when viewed from side
- Marked hourglass shape to waist when viewed from above
- No visible ventral fat pad

BCS 3 — IDEAL

- Ribs and spine palpable with slight pressure but not visible; no excess fat covering
- Good muscle tone apparent
- Concave abdominal tuck when viewed from side
- Hourglass shape to waist when viewed from above
- Minimal ventral fat pad palpable

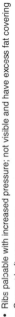

BCS 4
Overweight

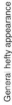

- Ribs palpable with increased pressure; not visible and have excess fat covering
- General hefty appearance
- Abdominal concave tuck is reduced or absent when viewed from the side
- Loss of hourglass shape to waist with back slightly widened when viewed from above
- Visible ventral fat pad

BCS 5
Obese

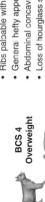

- Ribs and spine not palpable under a heavy fat covering
- Fat deposits visible over lumbar area, tail base, and spine
- Loss of hourglass shape to waist
- Complete loss of abdominal tuck
- Back is markedly widened
- Prominent ventral fat pad, which may sway from side to side when walking

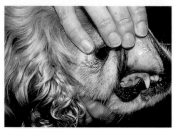

Icterus mucous membrane color in a cocker spaniel with liver disease.

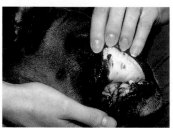

Pale mucous membrane in a boxer with a packed cell volume of 13%.

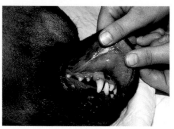

Brick-red mucous membrane in a mongrel with septic shock.

SOAP Progress Notes

	Component	Method	Examples
S	Subjective	Appearance	Panting, BAR, vocalizations
O	Objective	Physiologic data	TPR, presence of diarrhea, PCV, radiographic findings
A*	Assessment	Current status	Differential diagnosis
P*	Plan/Procedure	Next steps	Additional diagnostics, treatments, discharge

*Developed by the veterinarian.

COMMON VACCINATIONS FOR DOGS AND CATS

Cat Vaccines Licensed for Use in the United States[12A]

Vaccine Type	Recommended Interval	Minimum Duration of Immunity
Core Vaccines		
Panleukopenia: modified live (parenteral)	1 year following initial series, then every 3 years	7+ years

Continued

Cat Vaccines Licensed for Use in the United States[12A]—cont'd

Vaccine Type	Recommended Interval	Minimum Duration of Immunity
Herpesvirus-calicivirus: modified live (parenteral)	3 years	5+ years
Recombinant rabies (parenteral)	Annual	3 years
Rabies, 1-year: killed (parenteral)	Annual	3+ years
Rabies, 3-year: killed (parenteral)	3 years (as required by law)	3+ years
Noncore Vaccines		
Panleukopenia: killed (parenteral)	Annual	5+ years
Panleukopenia: modified live (topical)	3 years	Not known to be more than 1 year, but is likely
Herpesvirus-calicivirus: killed (parenteral)	Annual	5+ years
Herpesvirus-calicivirus: modified live (topical)	Annual (3-year duration of immunity is likely)	Not known, but expected to be at least 2 years
Chlamydophila felis: killed	Annual	1 year (maximum)
Chlamydophila felis: live, avirulent	Annual	

Recombinant feline leukemia	Annual	1 year
Feline leukemia virus: killed	Annual	1 year
Feline immunodeficiency virus: killed	Annual	1 year
Bordetella bronchiseptica: modified live (topical)	Annual	1 year

Dog Vaccines Licensed for Use in the United States[12A]

Vaccine Type	Recommended Interval	Minimum Duration of Immunity
Core Vaccines		
Distemper: modified live (parenteral)	3 years	5+ to 7+ years
Recombinant distemper (parenteral)	3 years	3+ years
Parvovirus: (modified live parenteral)	3 years	7+ years
Canine adenovirus-2: modified live (parenteral)	3 years	7+ years
Rabies 1 yr killed	1 year	
Rabies 3 yr killed	3 years	

Continued

Dog Vaccines Licensed for Use in the United States[12A]—cont'd

Vaccine Type	Recommended Interval	Minimum Duration of Immunity
Noncore Vaccines		
Distemper-measles: modified live (parenteral)	Not indicated	Not applicable
Parvovirus: killed (parenteral)	Annual	1 year
Canine adenovirus-2: killed (parenteral)	Annual	Unknown
Parainfluenza virus: modified live (parenteral)	3 years	5+ years
Parainfluenza virus: modified live (topical)	3 years	5+ years (preferred)
Bordetella bronchiseptica: killed (parenteral)	Annual	~12 months
Bordetella bronchiseptica: avirulent live (topical)	Annual	~12 months
Bordetella bronchiseptica: antigen extract (parenteral)	Annual	1 year

Leptospira var. canicola	Annual	Not definitively established (antibody titers persist for approximately 3 months in dogs that seroconvert after an initial vaccination series)
Leptospira var. icterhemorrhagiae	Annual	
Leptospira var. pomona	Annual	
Leptospira var. grippotyphosa	Annual	
Recombinant Lyme (parenteral)	Annual	1 year
Lyme: killed (parenteral)	Annual	1 year
Crotalus atrox (rattlesnake vaccine)	Annual or as recommended by manufacturer based on risk	Unknown (license is conditional at this writing)

Nutrient Guidelines for Wellness[*22]

Life Stage	Energy kcal ME/g	Protein	Fat	Fiber	Calcium Dry Matter	Phosphorus	Sodium
Dog							
Growth/reproduction	3.5-5.0	22-35	10-25	5 max	0.7-1.7	0.6-1.3	0.35-0.6
Large-breed growth	3.0-4.0	22-35	8-12	10 max	0.7-1.2	0.6-1.1	0.3-0.6
Adult maintenance	3.5-4.5	15-30	10-20	5 max	0.5-1.0	0.4-0.9	0.2-0.4
Obesity prone	3.0-3.5	15-30	7-12	5-17	0.5-1.0	0.4-0.9	0.2-0.4
High energy	>4.5	22-34	26 min	5 max	0.5-1.0	0.4-0.9	0.2-0.5
Geriatric[†]	3.5-4.5	15-23	7-15	10 max	0.5-1.0	0.2-0.7	0.15-0.35

Cat

Growth/reproduction	4.0-5.0	35-50	18-35	5 max	0.8-1.6	0.6-1.4	0.3-0.6
Adult maintenance	4.0-5.0	30-45	10-30	5 max	0.5-1.0	0.5-0.8	0.2-0.6
Obesity prone	3.3-3.8	30-45	8-17	5-15	0.5-1.0	0.5-0.9	0.2-0.6
Geriatric[+]	3.5-4.5	30-45	10-25	10 max	0.6-1.0	0.5-0.7	0.2-0.5

Max, Maximum; *min*, minimum; *C*, cup.

*Nutrients are expressed as % dry matter. Energy is expressed as kcal metabolizable energy (ME) per gram dry matter.

[+]Older animals require frequent body condition scoring. Feed intake adjustment may be required to maintain an ideal body condition because some older individuals tend to be heavy and others tend to lose weight.

Average Caloric Content of Pet Foods

Dog food (generic, private label, grocery)

Dry   350 kcal/C
Soft-moist   275 kcal/C
Canned   500 kcal/14- to 15-oz can

Cat food (generic, private label, grocery)

Dry   300 kcal/C
Soft-moist   250 kcal/C
Canned   180 kcal/5.5- to 6.5-oz can

Common Diseases of Dogs and Cats

Anal Saculitis

Causes: Impaction, inflammation, or infection of anal glands
Signs: Scooting, tail chewing, malodorous perinanal discharge

Anemia

Causes: Hemorrhage, iron deficiency, toxins, immune disorders
Signs: Anorexia, weakness, depression, tachycardia, tachypnea, pale mucous membranes

Arthritis

Causes: *Acute*—sepsis, trauma, immune-mediated; *Osteoarthritis*—progressive degeneration of hyaline cartilage
Signs: Lameness, swelling, crepitus

Asthma (Feline)

Causes: Inflammation of airways, broncho-constriction
Signs: Dyspnea (acute onset), coughing, lethargy

Atopy

Cause: Allergic reaction to inhaled substances
Signs: Pruritus, alopecia, dermatitis

Aural Hematoma

Cause: Trauma causing buildup of blood beneath skin surface
Signs: Head shaking, scratching at ear

Brachycephalic Respiratory Distress Syndrome

Cause: Congenital airway obstruction
Signs: Coughing, exercise intolerance, cyanosis, dyspnea

Common Diseases of Dogs and Cats—cont'd

Calicivirus (Feline)

Cause: Viral infection of upper respiratory tract
Signs: Anorexia, lethargy, fever, ulcerative stomatitis, nasal discharge

Cataracts

Causes: Inherited or secondary to diabetes and other diseases
Signs: Opaque pupillary opening, progressive vision loss

Congestive Heart Failure

Causes: Valvular insufficiency, myocarditis, hypertension, dilated cardiomyopathy
Signs: Anorexia, syncope, pulmonary edema

Coronavirus

Cause: Viral infection of gastrointestinal system
Signs: Asymptomatic or anorexia, dehydration, V/D

Cushing's Disease

Cause: Hyperadrenocorticism
Signs: Bilateral, symmetrical alopecia

Cystitis

Causes: Inflammation or bacterial infection of urinary bladder
Signs: Hematuria, dysuria, inappropriate urination, pollakuria, polyuria

Demodex

Cause: Infestation of hair follicles with *Demodex* mites
Signs: Alopecia, erythema, secondary pyoderma, pruritus

Continued

Common Diseases of Dogs and Cats—cont'd

Dermatophytosis

Causes: *Microsporum canis, M. gypseum,* or *Trichophyton mentagrophytes* infection
Signs: Circular area of alopecia; lesion may be raised, red, crusty

Diabetes Mellitus

Causes: Deficient or defective production of insulin
Signs: PU/PD, weight loss, polyphagia

Dilated Cardiomyopathy

Cause: Dilution of all chambers of the heart
Signs: Ascites, hepatomegaly, weight loss, abdominal distension, dyspnea

Distemper (Canine)

Cause: Paramyxoviral infection
Signs: Fever, cough, mucopurulent ocular and nasal discharge, V/D, hyperkeratosis of foot pads, ataxia

Dystocia

Causes: Primary uterine inertia, fetal obstruction
Signs: Active prolonged straining with no fetus produced, green, purulent, or hemorrhagic vaginal discharge, pain

Feline Fibrosarcoma

Cause: Vaccine-induced
Signs: Swelling and rapidly growing firm mass at site of recent vaccination

Flea Allergy Dermatitis

Cause: Hypersensitivity to *Ctenocephalides* infestation
Signs: Pruritus, licking, chewing, erythema, alopecia

Fungal Infection (Systemic)

Cause: *Blastomyces dermatidis*
Signs: Anorexia, depression, fever, dyspnea

Causes: *Coccidioides immitis*
Signs: Cough, fever, anorexia, weight loss

Causes: *Histoplasum capsulatum*
Signs: Weight loss, fever, anorexia

Geriatric Vestibular Syndrome

Cause: Otitis media
Signs: Head tilt, circling, disorientation, ataxia, nystagmus

Glaucoma

Cause: Increased intraocular fluid production
Signs: Ocular pain, corneal edema, buphthalmus, blindness

Heartworm Disease

Cause: *Dirofilaria immitis* parasite
Signs: Exercise intolerance (dogs), dyspnea, coughing, ascites (dogs), V (cats)

Hemobartonellosis

Cause: Mycoplasma rickettsial infection
Signs: Pale or icteric mucous membranes, fever, tachypnea, tachycardia

Hip Dysplasia

Cause: Laxity and subluxation of the hip joint
Signs: Lameness, gait abnormality, muscle atrophy

Histiocytoma

Cause: Benign skin tumor
Signs: Fast-growing dome or buttonlike nodules; may be ulcerated

Continued

Common Diseases of Dogs and Cats—cont'd

Hyperthyroidism

Cause: Overproduction of thyroid hormone
Signs: Weight loss, polyphagia, V, enlarged thyroid

Hypothyroidism

Cause: Underproduction of thyroid hormone
Signs: Weight gain, bilateral, symmetrical alopecia, cold intolerance

Hepatic Lipidosis

Cause: Accumulation of triglycerides in liver
Signs: Prolonged anorexia, V/D, lethargy

Immune-Mediated Hemolytic Anemia

Cause: Accelerated red blood cell destruction
Signs: Anorexia, depression, tachycardia, tachypnea, pale mucous membranes

Immunodeficiency Virus (Feline)

Cause: Lentivirus infection
Signs: Chronic infections of oral cavity, skin, respiratory tract, etc.; chronic fever, cachexia

Infectious Canine Tracheobronchitis (Kennel Cough)

Causes: Bacterial and viral infection of lower respiratory tract (*Bordatella bronchiseptica*, canine adenovirus, etc.)
Signs: Dry, hacking, paroxysmal cough

Inflammatory Bowel Disease

Cause: Inflammation of intestinal mucosa
Signs: D, increased frequency and volume of defecation

Common Diseases of Dogs and Cats—cont'd

Intestinal Parasitism

Causes: Infection with parasites including nematodes (i.e., ascarids, hookworms, whipworms, etc.), coccidia, protozoa (i.e., *Giardia*), cestodes, etc.

Signs: Depending on species of parasite; D, weight loss, anemia, unthriftiness

Lipoma

Cause: Benign fatty tumor

Signs: Soft and round or oval subcuticular mass

Liver Disease

Causes: Drugs, toxins, bile duct inflammation

Signs: Anorexia, V/D, PU/PD, jaundice

Lyme Disease

Cause: *Borrelia burgdorferi*

Signs: Fever, anorexia, lameness, lymphadenopathy

Osteochondrosis dessicans

Cause: Degeneration and reossification of bone and cartilage

Signs: Lameness, crepitus, pain

Otitis Externa

Causes: Primary or secondary parasitic, bacterial, or yeast infection of the soft tissues of the ear

Signs: Head shaking, head tilt, pain, foul odor

Panleukoponia (Feline)

Cause: Parvoviral infection

Signs: Anorexia, fever, V/D, abdominal pain

Continued

Common Diseases of Dogs and Cats—cont'd

Panosteitis

Causes: Possible viral infection, metabolic disease, allergic reaction, hormonal excesses
Signs: Intermittent lameness, anorexia, fever, weight loss

Pancreatitis

Cause: Inflammation of the pancreas due to obesity, overingestion of fats, other diseases
Signs: Depression, anorexia, V/D, dehydration

Parvovirus (Canine)

Cause: Viral infection of gastrointestinal tract
Signs: Bloody D, lethargy, V, dehydration, fever

Patella Luxation

Causes: Genetic predisposition, trauma
Signs: Abnormal gait with rotation of limbs

Periodontal Disease

Cause: Bacterial infection of tissues surrounding teeth that leads to plaque accumulation and causes calculus buildup
Signs: Increased depth of periodontal pockets, increased tooth mobility, foul oral odor, pain

Peritonitis

Cause: Inflammatory process
Signs: Abdominal pain, reluctance to move, tachycardia, tachypnea, fever, V/D, dehydration

Pyoderma (Deep)

Cause: Bacterial infection of the skin usually caused by *Staphylococcus intermedius*
Signs: Papules, pustules, draining fistulous tracts

Common Diseases of Dogs and Cats—cont'd

Pyometra

Cause: Bacterial infection (*E. coli, Staphylococcus, Pasteurella,* etc.)
Signs: Vulvar discharge, abdominal enlargement, PU/PD, dehydration

Renal Failure

Cause: Damage to nephron causing reduction in glomerular filtration
Signs: Oliguria, polyuria, V/D, anorexia, dehydration

Sarcoptic Mange

Cause: *Scabies scabei* mite infestation
Signs: Red, crusty lesions; intense pruritus

Skin Tumors (Sebaceous Cysts, Adenoma, Adenocarcinoma, Melanoma)

Causes: Unknown; possible genetic causes
Signs: Usually round masses, may be encapsulated or ulcerated

Thrombocytopenia

Causes: Numerous viral, bacterial, immune-mediated and other noninfectious causes
Signs: Petechial hemorrhage, ecchymosis, epistaxis, lethargy

Tick-Borne Rickettsial Disease

Causes: *Rickettsia rickettsii* (Rocky Mountain spotted fever)
Signs: Fever, anorexia, mucopurulent ocular discharge, coughing, tachypnea, V/D
Causes: *Ehrlichia canis, E. ewingi, E. equi* (ehrlichiosis)
Signs: Lymphadenopathy, anemia, depression, anorexia, fever lethargy, lameness, muscular stiffness

Continued

Common Diseases of Dogs and Cats—cont'd

Ulcerative Keratitis (Corneal Ulcers)

Causes: Trauma, bacterial infection, feline herpesvirus
Signs: Ocular pain, corneal edema, photophobia

Urolithiasis

Cause: Precipitation of mineral substances in urine
Signs: Dysuria, hematuria

Viral Rhinotracheitis (Feline)

Cause: Herpesvirus infection
Signs: Acute onset of sneezing, conjunctivitis, purulent rhinitis, fever

von Willebrand's Disease

Cause: Decreased or deficient production of von Willebrand's factor
Signs: Purpura, prolonged bleeding from venipuncture or surgical sites

Viral Enteritis

Causes: Parvovirus, coronavirus, rotavirus feline
Signs: Bloody D, lethargy, V, dehydration, fever

D, Diarrhea; *PD,* polydypsia; *PU,* polyuria; *V,* vomiting.

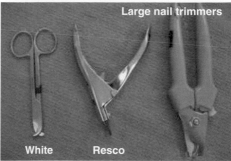

Large nail trimmers

White   Resco

Nail trimmers are available in a variety of styles and sizes. Guillotine-type trimmers (Resco) are available in regular and large sizes. The blade can be replaced when it becomes dull. Scissors-type trimmers (White) work well for ingrown nails, for nails of puppies and kittens, and for cat claws. The trimmers must always be clean and sharp.

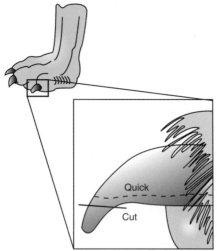

All types of trimmer blades are positioned within 2 mm from the end of the quick. With a swift, smooth motion, the nail is cut just distal to the quick. In patients with white nails, the quick is visible and easy to avoid. In those with dark nails, the end of the nail is pared down a little at a time until a clearer or lighter color appears in the cross section of the nail. This is the tip of the quick. The remaining untrimmed dark nails are compared with the trimmed nail for proper length of trim.

▰▰ EXPRESSING ANAL SACS[23] ▰▰

Anatomy of the canine anal sacs are located at approximately the 4 o'clock and 8 o'clock positions. The anal sacs are best emptied, or "expressed," using the internal technique of inserting a lubricated, gloved forefinger into the rectum. External expression of the anal sacs is a technique that requires squeezing the anal glands from the external anal sphincter.

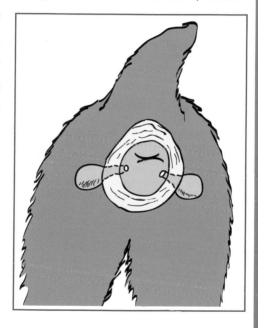

MATERIALS

- Basin
- Bulb syringe
- Cotton balls or cotton swabs
- Hemostats
- Ceruminolytic agents, saline solution, cleansing
- Solution or dilute vinegar

PROCEDURE

1. Tip the head and ear slightly ventrally, grasp the pinna, and place the solution into the ear canal with the bulb syringe directed ventromedially into the canal. Have the basin ready below the ear to catch the excess.

2. Massage the base of the ear to distribute the cleansing solution and to loosen any debris. Flush the ear again. Use cotton balls on a hemostat to clean the debris in the ear canal. Never insert cotton-tipped swabs into the canal of an inadequately restrained patient. Use cotton swabs for the external ear canal and interior of the pinna only. Allow the patient to shake its head occasionally to loosen more debris. Flush and clean the ears until debris is no longer visible. Dry the ear canal with cotton balls.

3. Examine the ears with an otoscope, and apply any medications necessary. Massage the ear canal to distribute the medication evenly and thoroughly.

AGE EQUIVALENTS FOR DOGS[29]

Comparative Age in Human Years

Dog's Age	0-20 lbs	21-50 lbs	51-90 lbs	>90 lbs
5 years	36	37	40	42
6 years	40	42	45	49
7 years	44	47	50	56
10 years	56	60	66	78
12 years	64	69	77	93
15 years	76	83	93	115
20 years	96	105	120	—

AGE EQUIVALENTS FOR CATS[29]

Cat's Age	Comparative Age in Human Years
1 year	15
2 years	24
5 years	36
7 years	45
12 years	64
15 years	76
18 years	88
21 years	100

DIAGNOSTIC AND TREATMENT
TECHNIQUES

DIAGNOSTIC IMAGING

ADMINISTERING OTIC AND OPHTHALMIC MEDICATIONS[28]

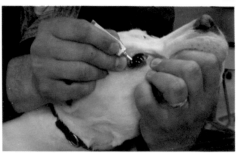

Turn the dog's head toward the person administering the drug with both hands around the head or a hand around the muzzle.

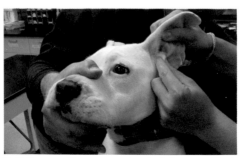

Pull the ear pinna up and out of the way. Tuck the ear over the dog's head, and position it between the head and the examiner's body.

Procedures

INJECTION TECHNIQUES[22]

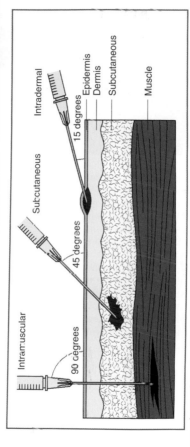

Comparison of angle of injection and location of medication deposit for IM, SQ, and ID injections.

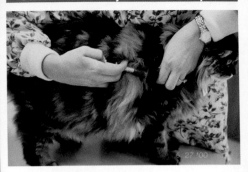

1. Grasp the skin between thumb and fore-finger along the dorsolateral aspect of the neck or back and lift gently to form a tent.
   a. Avoid intrascapular area, especially for vaccines and insulin administration.
2. Insert the needle into the skin fold and aspirate.
   a. If blood is aspirated, withdraw the needle and use another injection site.
   b. If no blood is aspirated, inject the medication or fluids slowly.
3. Multiple injection sites can be used along the dorsum and lateral to the spine.

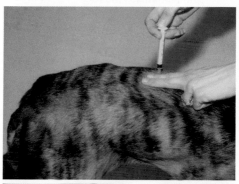

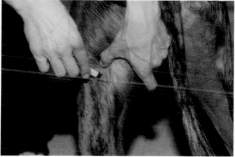

1. Ensure patient is properly restrained.
2. Locate muscle group of choice by palpation.
   a. Epaxial muscles lateral to the dorsal spinous process of lumbar vertebrae 3 to 5.
   b. Quadriceps muscles of the cranial thigh.
   c. Triceps muscles caudal to the humerus.

    d. Lateral aspect of semimembranosus/
       semitendinosus muscles.
3. Swab the injection site with a disinfectant.
4. Insert the needle 1 to 2 cm at a 45- to
   90-degree angle.
5. Aspirate the syringe to ensure the needle
   is not placed in a blood vessel.
    a. If blood is aspirated, withdraw the
      needle and insert into a different site.
    b. If no blood is aspirated, inject the medi-
      cation at a slow to moderate rate.
6. Remove the needle and massage the
   muscle to disperse the medication.

Intradermal Injection Technique

1. Shave the hair from a large area over the
   lateral thorax or abdomen.
2. Wipe the skin carefully with water-
   moistened gauze.
3. Hold the skin taut between the thumb and
   forefinger of the left hand and insert the
   needle (bevel up) into the skin at an angle
   of approximately 10 degrees into the der-
   mis.
4. Inject a small amount of material to form a
   wheal (bleb) at the site.
    a. If no bleb forms, the injection may
      have been subcutaneous and not intra-
      dermal.

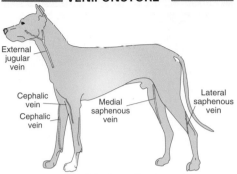

External
jugular
vein

Cephalic
vein

Cephalic
vein

Medial
saphenous
vein

Lateral
saphenous
vein

The veins accessible for collection of venous blood in dogs and cats.

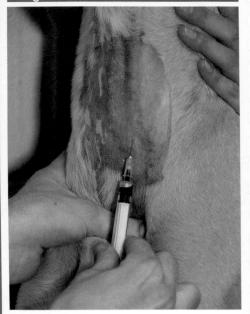

1. Clip hair from a small area over the jugular furrow.
2. Distend the vein with blood (raise the vein) by applying firm pressure at the thoracic inlet at the most ventral portion of the jugular furrow, lateral to the trachea.
3. Palpate the distended vein.
4. Apply alcohol and allow alcohol to dry.
5. Insert the needle, bevel upward, at a 20- to 30-degree angle to the vein.

6. Once the tip of the needle is in the vein, apply suction to collect the sample or insert vacutainer tube onto collection needle.

7. Once the sample is collected, release the pressure on the vein, halt suction, and withdraw the needle from the vein.

8. Place gentle pressure on the venipuncture site, and hold for approximately 60 seconds.

Cephalic Blood Collection Procedure[32]

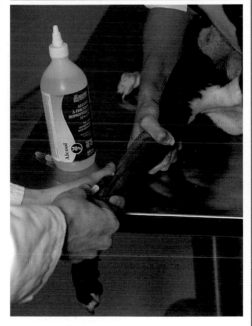

1. Restrain the patient in a sitting position or in sternal recumbency.
2. Clip hair from a small area over the dorsal forelimb.
3. Swab the site with alcohol and allow the alcohol to dry.
4. Have a restrainer occlude the vessel, by placing the thumb on the medial aspect of the limb, compressing down with the thumb and rolling the hand laterally.
   a. The restrainer should stand on the side opposite the leg to be used, and should use one arm to restrain the animal's head by encircling the neck and turning the muzzle away from the leg to be used.
   b. The restrainer should use the other arm to extend the animal's front leg by holding the elbow and pushing the leg forward.
5. Grasp the paw to keep the leg extended.
6. Identify the distended cephalic vein and place the thumb alongside the vein to stabilize it during venipuncture.
7. Insert the needle, bevel upward, at a 20- to 30-degree angle to the vein.
8. Once the tip of the needle is in the vein, apply suction to collect the sample.
9. Once the sample is collected, have the holder release the pressure on the vein.
10. Halt suction and withdraw the needle from the vein.
11. Place gentle pressure on the venipuncture site, and hold for approximately 60 seconds.

Lateral Saphenous Blood Collection[32]

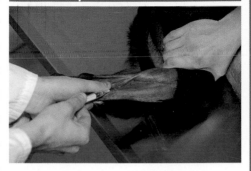

1. Clip hair from a small area over the vein.
2. Have the animal restrained in lateral recumbency with the legs toward the venipuncturist and the back toward the holder.
   a. Restrain by grasping the forelimbs with one hand and elevating them slightly off the table while applying pressure down on the neck of the patient with the same forearm.
3. Grasp the uppermost hind leg with the other hand.
4. Grasp the hind foot and palpate the distended vein.
5. Swab the area over the vein with alcohol and allow the alcohol to dry.
6. Place the thumb adjacent to the vein to stabilize it and prevent movement during venipuncture.
7. Insert the needle, bevel upward, at a 20- to 30-degree angle to the vein.
8. Once the tip of the needle is in the vein, apply suction to collect the sample.

9. Once the sample is collected, release the pressure on the vein, halt suction, and withdraw the needle from the vein.
10. Place gentle pressure on the venipuncture site, and hold for approximately 60 seconds.

Medial Saphenous Blood Collection Procedure[32]

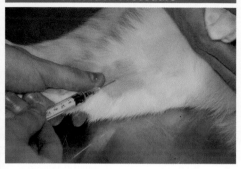

1. Clip a small amount of hair from the area over the vein.
2. Have the animal restrained in lateral recumbency with the legs toward the venipuncturist and the back toward the holder.
   a. The restrainer should hold the animal's head with one hand while retracting the uppermost hind leg with the other hand.
   b. The restrainer applies pressure in the inguinal region to occlude the medial saphenous vein and cause it to distend with blood.

3. Grasp the metatarsal region of the rear limb closest to the table and extend the leg.
4. Palpate the distended vein.
5. Place the thumb adjacent to the vein to stabilize it and prevent movement during venipuncture.
6. Insert the needle, bevel upward, into the vein.
7. Once the tip of the needle is in the vein, apply very slight suction to collect the sample.
8. Once the sample is collected, have the holder release pressure on the vein.
9. Halt suction and withdraw the needle from the vein.
10. Place gentle pressure on the venipuncture site, and hold for approximately 60 seconds.

CAST APPLICATION[23]

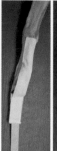 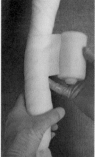 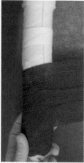

Place tape stirrups on the lateral aspects of the limb. Place a tongue depressor between them to prevent adherence of the stirrups to each other. Apply a stockinette over the limb and then a lightly padded, secondary layer firmly around the leg. Apply the fiberglass casting material firmly but not tightly to the leg, taking care to avoid compression of the cast material with the fingers. Bivalve the cast by cutting it lengthwise. This reduces the risk of excessive compression of the leg. Tape the two halves together, reflect the stockinette ends over the cast, and reflect the tape stirrups onto the cast. Apply protective tape over the cast. The caudal half of the cast can be used alone as a custom-fitted splint.

ROBERT JONES BANDAGE[23]

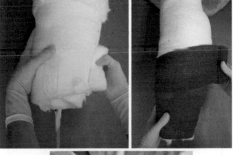

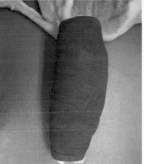

Apply tape stirrups, and wrap the limb in a secondary layer of roll cotton that extends beyond the joints above and below the fracture or injury. Compress the roll cotton tightly with a conforming gauze layer. Avoid excessive twisting of the leg as the gauze layer is tightened. Reflect the stirrups on top of the gauze. Apply protective tape (nonocclusive) firmly. The completed bandage should feel solid, and a "ping" should be heard on percussion.

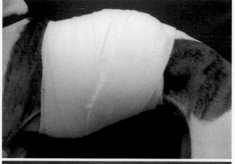

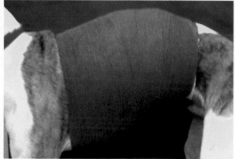

After a primary layer is placed on the wound, the padded secondary layer is applied. This is followed by application of a gauze tertiary layer. Protective tape is then applied.

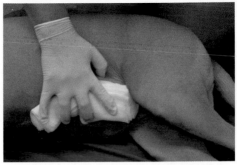

In the initial step of applying an abdominal pressure bandage, folded gauze is placed on midline to provide a padded site of pressure.

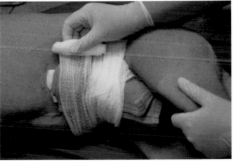

A rolled towel may be placed on top of the gauze pad to add to the cushion and further focus the bandage pressure. Gauze cling is used to secure the bandage material on midline and apply appropriate tension. Additional layers of bandage material are applied to secure the bandage.

Lavage Solutions[38]

Cleanser	Advantage	Disadvantage
Tap water	Availability Inexpensive Ease of application	Hypotonic Cytotoxic trace elements Not antimicrobial
Balanced electrolyte solution: Lactated Ringer's solution (LRS), Normosol	Isotonic Least cytotoxic	Not antimicrobial
Normal (0.9%) solution	Isotonic	Slightly more acidic than LRS Not antimicrobial
0.05% Chlorhexidine (1 part stock solution to 40 parts sterile water or LRS or (≈25 ml stock solution per liter)	Wide antimicrobial spectrum Good residual activity Not inactivated by organic matter	Precipitates in electrolyte solutions More concentrated solutions are cytotoxic and may slow granulation tissue formation *Proteus*, *Pseudomonas*, and *Candida* are resistant Corneal toxicity

0.1% Povidone-iodine (1 part stock to 100 parts LRS) or (≈10 ml stock to 100 ml LRS)	Wide antimicrobial spectrum	Inactivated by organic matter Limited residual activity Cytotoxic at concentrations greater than 1% Contact hypersensitivity Thyroid disorders if absorbed

Feeding Tubes[1]

Duration	Advantages	Disadvantages
Nasoesophageal (NE) Tube		
Short term (<5 days)	Inexpensive, easy to place, no anesthesia required.	Requires liquid diet. Some animals will not eat with NE tube in place.
Esophagostomy (E) Tube		
Long term	Inexpensive. Easy to place. Can use with calorie-dense diets.	Requires anesthsia. Cellulitis can occur if tube is removed too early.
Gastrostomy (G) Tube*		
Long term	Easy to place.	Requires anesthesia.
Percutaneous Endoscopically Guided (PEG) Tube		
Long term	Can use with calorie-dense diets.	Requires endoscope.
Surgically Placed		
Long term	Can use with calorie-dense diets.	Requires anesthesia and laparotomy.
Jejunostomy (J) Tube		
Long term	Bypasses stomach and pancreas. Can be used in patients with pancreatitis.	Requires anesthesia and laparatomy for all in-hospital use. Requires continuous rate infusion. Requires liquid diet. Peritonitis can occur if tube is removed.

*For all G tubes, peritonitis is a possible complication if the tube leaks or is removed too early.

■■■■ EMERGENCY SUPPLIES[12] ■■■■

- Laryngoscope (various size blades)
- Endotracheal tubes (various sizes)
- Cotton roll gauze to tie in endotracheal tube
- Stylette for intubation
- Rigid catheter (tomcat and long urinary) to assist with intubation and endotracheal drug administration
- 3-, 6-, and 12-ml syringes taken out of case and attached to 22-gauge needles
- 22-gauge needles
- Ambubag and oxygen source
- Electrocardiogram monitor
- Epinephrine
- Atropine
- Naloxone
- Calcium gluconate or calcium chloride
- Magnesium chloride
- Amiodarone
- 0.9% saline
- 50% dextrose
- Laceration pack for slash tracheostomy
- Intravenous catheters
- 1-inch white tape
- Emergency drug table with dose and volume and route of administration for various size animals

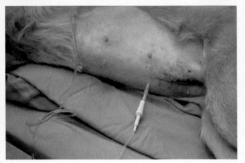

Sterile saline is injected into the abdomen via a catheter or needle and allowed to mix with abdominal contents before abdominocentesis.

DIAGNOSTIC PERITONEAL LAVAGE

Materials

- Peritoneal lavage catheter or over-the-needle catheter
- Lactated Ringer's solution or normal saline
- Intravenous (IV) administration and/or extension sets
- Surgical kit
- Sterile gloves
- Laboratory collection tubes

Procedure

1. Empty the bladder and clip and prepare the skin caudal to the umbilicus.
2. Infiltrate the skin and abdominal wall with lidocaine.
3. Make a small incision through the skin, subcutaneous tissue, and superficial abdominal fascia.

4. Insert the catheter through the incision, and direct it caudally and dorsally.
5. Infuse 20 ml/kg of warmed lactated Ringer's solution or normal saline into the abdomen. Gently rock the patient from side-to-side for a few minutes.
6. Collect the fluid aseptically as it flows freely from the catheter; fluid removal may require gentle aspiration.
7. Remove the catheter if the fluid is clear. Otherwise, suture it in place and use as needed.
8. If necessary, perform gross, cytologic, and biochemical analysis on the sample.

CARDIOPULMONARY RESUSCITATION[23]

CARDIOPULMONARY RESUSCITATION (CPR) PROCEDURE

1. **Extend the head and neck** to create an airway.
2. **Open the jaws** to check for obstructions.
3. **Cup your hands around the muzzle** of the dog's mouth so that only the nostrils are clear. Blow air into the nostrils with five or six quick breaths. Continue at a rate of 12 to 20 breaths per minute.
4. **Perform chest compressions:** Place both hands, palms down, between the third and sixth ribs on the chest cavity.
5. **Use the heels of your hands** to push down for 10 to 15 quick compressions (3 compressions every 6 seconds)
6. **Give the dog two breaths of air** in the nostrils after each cycle of compression.

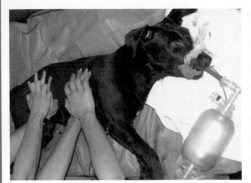

Appropriate hand placement for chest compressions. Also note placement of hands for abdominal compressions.

CPR[23]

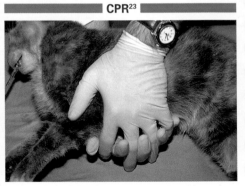

Placement of the hands in an animal less than 15 pounds is essential for the administration of chest compression, which simulates cardiac contractions (the cardiac pump).

Catheter Selection[4]

Patient Size (in Pounds)	Vein	Type of Catheter	Catheter Diameter (Gauge)
Canine			
0-5	Saphenous/cephalic	Over the needle	24
5-25	Saphenous/cephalic	Over the needle	22
25-80	Saphenous/cephalic	Over the needle	20
80 and up	Saphenous/cephalic	Over the needle	18
0-5	Jugular	Through the needle	21
5-25	Jugular	Through the needle	18
25-80	Jugular	Through the needle	16-18
80 and up	Jugular	Through the needle	16
0-5	Saphenous/cephalic	Butterfly	24-23
5-25	Saphenous/cephalic	Butterfly	22
25-80	Saphenous/cephalic	Butterfly	20
80 and up	Saphenous/cephalic	Butterfly	18
Feline			
0-4	Femoral/cephalic	Over the needle	24
4 and up	Femoral/cephalic	Over the needle	22
0-4	Jugular	Through the needle	21
4 and up	Jugular	Through the needle	18
0-4	Cephalic	Butterfly	24
4 and up	Cephalic	Butterfly	22

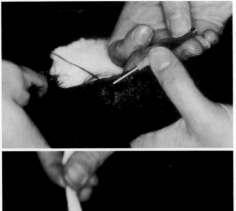

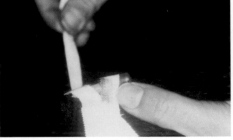

Place an over-the-needle catheter in the cephalic vein of a dog. Slide the catheter off the stylet into the vein as soon as blood is present in the needle hub. Place a cap on the end of the catheter immediately after it is completely inserted into the vein. Keep the catheter in place by wrapping several strips of tape around the catheter and circumference of the front leg. Press the thumb against the catheter cap to prevent the catheter from backing out of the vein as it is taped.

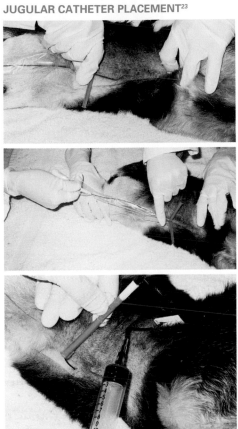

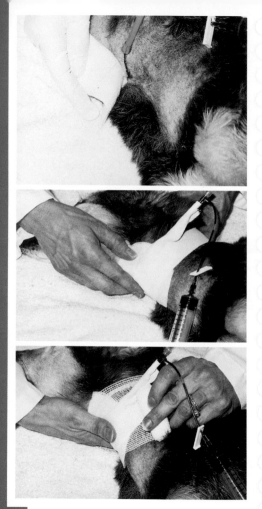

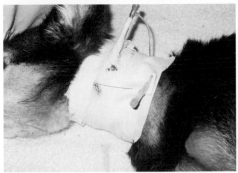

The needle (with blue plastic guard folded back) is inserted through skin just lateral to the left jugular vein. The catheter is fed into the vein through a protective plastic sleeve. Once the needle has been removed from the vein, the plastic guard is folded back over the needle. The catheter remains in the vein and exits the skin through the needle. The patency of the catheter is checked by aspirating blood through the syringe. Antibiotic ointment is placed on a gauze sponge and applied to the catheter entry site. Tape is placed along the needle guard and is wrapped over the gauze sponge and the circumference of the neck. Roll gauze is used to secure the catheter to the neck. As a final step, the gauze wrap is covered with waterproof tape.

FLUID THERAPY

CALCULATION OF FLUID REQUIREMENTS[22]

Body weight (kg) × % dehydration × 1000 = ml fluid deficit*

(60 to 80 ml/kg) × Body weight (kg) = ml of daily fluid requirement*

Estimation of ongoing losses × 2 = ml of ongoing losses*

Example: 20 kg dog, 8% dehydrated, 100 ml vomitus

20 kg × 0.08 1000 = 1600 ml

(20 kg) × (60 mg/kg) = 1200 ml

100 ml × 2 = 200 ml

Total volume = 3000 ml/24 = 125 ml/hr

	15 Drops/ml		60 Drops/ml	
ml/hr	drops/min	sec-drops	drops/min	sec-drops
5	—	—	5	12
10	—	—	10	6
15	—	—	15	4
20	—	—	20	3
25	—	—	25	2
30	—	—	30	2
35	—	—	35	2
40	10	6	40	2
45	11	5	45	1.5
50	12	5	50	1
55	14	4	55	1
60	15	4	60	—
65	16	4	—	—

Intravenous Fluid Rate Calculations[1]

Continued

	Intravenous Fluid Rate Calculations[1]— cont'd			
	15 Drops/ml		**60 Drops/ml**	
ml/hr	drops/ min	sec- drops	drops/ min	sec-drops
70	18	3	—	—
75	19	3	—	—
80	20	3	—	—
85	21	3	—	—
90	23	3	—	—
95	24	2.5	—	—
100	25	2	—	—
125	31	2	—	—
150	38	1.5	—	—

MONITORING FLUID THERAPY

- Note presence or absence of ocular or nasal discharge
- Evaluate for presence of chemosis, subcutaneous edema
- Auscultate lung sounds
- Note respiratory rate and effort
- Evaluate for presence of coughing, restlessness
- Measure central venous pressure
- Monitor urine output

CENTRAL VENOUS PRESSURE[23]

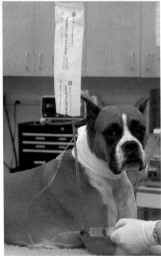

Central venous pressure measurement using a manometer connected to a central line catheter can be used to monitor hydration status and response to fluid therapy.

TONOMETRY[31]

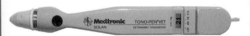

The Tono-Pen measures intraocular pressure (IOP). The end of this instrument is placed on the surface of the eye, which engages a pressure plate that measures the ocular pressure of the eye. The pressure is displayed in a digital window. Normal IOP in dogs and cats is 10 to 20 mm Hg.

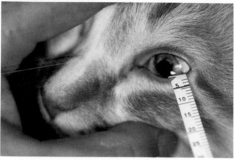

Schirmer tear test strip in position.

Normal Schirmer Tear Test Values (mm/min)[20]

Species	No. 1	Low, but Disease Usually Not Present	Abnormal	No. 2
Dog	19.8 ± 5.3	5-11*	<5	11.6 ± 6.1
Cat	16.9 ± 5.7	5-11	<5	—
Horse	>15	10-15	<10	—
Cow	>15	10-15	<10	—
Rabbit	5.3 ± 2.96	—	—	—

*Some dogs will show clinical signs between 10 and 14 mm. The breed and history of signs consistent with intermittent keratoconjunctivitis sicca are useful in determining a diagnosis.

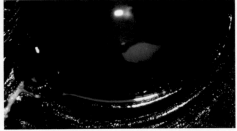

Characteristic staining pattern of a superficial ulcer. Fluorescein stain adheres only to the floor of the ulcer and has distinct margins.

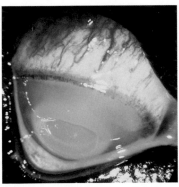

Characteristic staining pattern of a deeper stromal ulcer. Fluorescein stain adheres to the walls and floor of the ulcer. Some diffusion of fluorescein exists in the neighboring stroma.

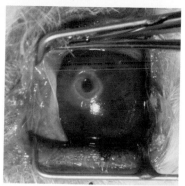

Characteristic staining pattern of a descemetocele. Fluorescein stain adheres only to the walls of the ulcer. The center of the ulcer fails to take up stain and appears black.

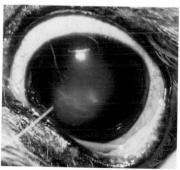

Characteristic staining pattern of an indolent ulcer. Fluorescein stains the floor of the ulcer but this area does not have distinct margins.

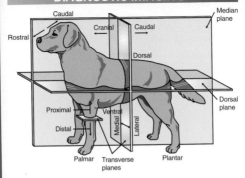

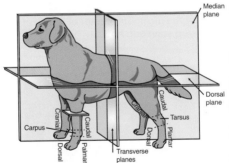

Anatomical planes of reference and directional terms.

Variable kV Technique Chart for an X-Ray Machine of 300 mA, 125 kV, 1/120-Second Timer with FFD of 40 Inches					
Thickness (cm)	**kV**	**mA**	**Seconds**	**mAs**	**Grid a:1**
4	48	300	1/120	2.5	No
5	50	300	1/120	2.5	No
6	52	300	1/120	2.5	No
7	54	300	1/120	2.5	No
8	56	300	1/120	2.5	No
9	58	300	1/120	2.5	No
10	63	300	1/60	5.0	Yes
11	65	300	1/60	5.0	Yes
12	67	300	1/60	5.0	Yes
13	69	300	1/60	5.0	Yes
14	71	300	1/60	5.0	Yes
15	73	300	1/60	5.0	Yes
16	75	300	1/60	5.0	Yes
17	77	300	1/60	5.0	Yes
18	79	300	1/60	5.0	Yes
19	81	300	1/60	5.0	Yes
20	84	300	1/60	5.0	Yes
21	87	300	1/60	5.0	Yes
22	90	300	1/60	5.0	Yes
23	93	300	1/60	5.0	Yes
24	96	300	1/60	5.0	Yes
25	99	300	1/60	5.0	Yes
26	102	300	1/60	5.0	Yes
27	105	300	1/60	5.0	Yes

Continued

Variable kV Technique Chart for an X-Ray Machine of 300 mA, 125 kV, 1/120-Second Timer with FFD of 40 Inches—cont'd

Thickness (cm)	kV	mA	Seconds	mAs	Grid a:1
28	99	300	1/30	10.0	Yes
29	102	300	1/30	10.0	Yes
30	105	300	1/30	10.0	Yes

FFD, Focal-film distance; *kV,* kilovolts; *mA,* milliamperes; *mAs,* milliamperes per second.

Radiographs were taken with Kodak Lanex Regular screens and Kodak TML x-ray film.

TROUBLESHOOTING IMAGE QUALITY ERRORS[23A]

INCREASED FILM DENSITY
- Too high mAs or kV settings
- Too short focal-film distance
- Wrong measurement of anatomic part

DECREASED FILM DENSITY
- Too low mAs or kV settings
- Too long focal-film distance
- Wrong measurement of anatomic part

BLACK MARKS OR ARTIFACTS
- Film scratches
- Static electricity (linear dots or tree pattern)
- Defective cassette (does not close properly)

WHITE MARKS (ARTIFACTS)
- Dirt or debris between the film and screen
- Defect or crack in screen
- Contrast medium on tabletop, skin, or cassette

GRAY FILM
- Film accidentally exposed to radiation (scattered, secondary, or direct)
- Lack of grid for examination of a thick part
- Outdated film
- Film stored in too hot or too humid place

DISTORTED OR BLURRED RADIOGRAPH
- Motion: patient, cassette, or machine
- Too great focal-film distance
- Poor film-screen contact

LINEAR ARTIFACTS
- Grid out of focal range
- Primary beam not centered
- Grid upside down or damaged

INCREASED FILM DENSITY
- Film overdeveloped
- Temperature of solution too high
- Wrong concentration of developer

DECREASED FILM DENSITY
- Film underdeveloped
- Temperature of solution too low
- Exhausted or contaminated developer
- Developer too diluted or improperly mixed

FOGGED FILMS
- Light leakage in darkroom
- Film exposed to radiation from any source
- Overdeveloped film
- Contaminated developer

YELLOW RADIOGRAPH
- Fixation time too short
- Exhausted fixer solution

WHITE SPOTS
- Defective screens: pitted, scratched
- Dust or grit on surface of film
- Fixer on film before processing

BLACK SPOTS
- Drops of developer solution on film before processing
- Films stacked together in fixer

BRITTLE RADIOGRAPHS
- Drying temperature too high
- Drying time too long

MISCELLANEOUS MISTAKES
- Film wet: too short drying time
- Grit on films: dirty tanks and solutions
- Corner marks: wet or dirty fingers on hangers
- Sticky film: film washed or dried improperly
- Static electricity: low humidity and rough or too fast handling of films
- Scratches: careless handling

Landmarks[29]

Cranial or Proximal Landmark	Caudal or Distal Landmark	Center Landmark	Comments
Thorax			
Manubrium sterni	Halfway between xiphoid and last rib	Heart	Expose at peak inspiration
Abdomen			
Three rib spaces cranial to xyphoid	Greater trochanter	Last rib	Expose at peak expiration
Shoulder			
Midbody scapula	Midshaft humerus	Over joint space	
Humerus			
Shoulder joint	Elbow joint	Midshaft	

Continued

Landmarks[29]—cont'd

Cranial or Proximal Landmark	Caudal or Distal Landmark	Center Landmark	Comments
Elbow			
Midshaft humerus	Midshaft radius	Over joint space	
Radius and Ulna			
Elbow joint	Carpal joint	Midshaft	
Carpus			
Midshaft radius	Midshaft metacarpus	Over joint space	
Metacarpus			
Carpal joint	Include digits	Midshaft	
Pelvis			
Wings of ilium	Ischium		

Pelvis Ventrodorsal View, Flexed				
Wings of ilium	Ischium			Pushes stifles cranially
Pelvis Ventrodorsal View, Extended				
Wings of ilium	Ischium			Femora parallel to each other and table
Femur				
Coxofemoral joint	Stifle joint	Tarsal joint		
Stifle				
Midshaft femur	Midshaft tibia	Over joint space		
Tibia and Fibula				
Stifle joint	Tarsal joint	Midshaft		
Tarsus				
Midshaft tibia	Midshaft metatarsal	Over joint space		

Continued

Landmarks[29]—cont'd

Cranial or Proximal Landmark	Caudal or Distal Landmark	Center Landmark	Comments
Metatarsus			
	Include digits	Midshaft	
Cervical Vertebrae			
Base of skull	Spine of scapula		Extend front limbs caudally, collimate width of beam to increase detail
Thoracic Vertebrae			
Spine of scapula	Halfway between xiphoid and last rib		Collimate width of beam to increase detail

Thoracolumbar Vertebrae		
	Halfway between xiphoid and last rib	Collimate width of beam to increase detail

Lumbar Vertebrae		
Halfway between xiphoid and last rib	Wings of ilium	Collimate width of beam to increase detail

Contrast Media[14]

Trade Name	Generic Name	Iodine (mg/ml)
Barium Liquid E-X Paque	Barium sulfate suspension 60%	—
Novopaque	Barium sulfate suspension 60%	—
BIPS	Barium-impregnated-polyethylene spheres	—
Gastrografin	Sodium diatrizoate and meglumine diatrizoate	367
Hypaque sodium 50%	Sodium diatrizoate 50%	300
Hypaque meglumine 60%	Meglumine diatrizoate 60%	282
Renografin 60	Sodium diatrizoate 8% and meglumine diatrizoate 52%	292
Renografin 76	Sodium diatrizoate 10% and meglumine diatrizoate 66%	370
Conray 60	Meglumine iothalamate 60%	282
Conray 325	Sodium iothalamate 66.8%	235
Isovue-M 200	Iopamidol	200
Omnipaque 240	Iohexol	240
Omnipaque 18	Iohexol	180
Radiopaque	Iohexol	200, 300, or 350
Visipaque 320	Iodixanol	320
Visipaque 270	Iodixanol	270
Magnevist	Gadolinium	—

DENTAL FORMULAS FOR CATS AND DOGS[29]

CATS
Deciduous: $2 \times (3i/3i, 1c/1c, 3p/2p) = 26$
Permanent: $2 \times (3I/3I, 1C/1C, 3P/2P, 1M/1M) = 30$

Time of Eruption		
	Deciduous	**Permanent**
Incisors	2 to 3 weeks	3 to 4 months
Canines	3 to 4 weeks	4 to 5 months
Premolars	3 to 6 weeks	4 to 6 months
Molars		4 to 6 months

DOGS
Deciduous: $2 \times (3i/3i, 1c/1c, 3p/2p) = 28$
Permanent: $2 \times (3I/3I, 1C/1C, 4P/4P, 2M/3M) = 42$

Time of Eruption		
	Deciduous	**Permanent**
Incisors	3 to 5 weeks	3 to 5 months
Canines	3 to 6 weeks	3.5 to 6 months
Premolars	4 to 10 weeks	3.5 to 6 months
Molars		3.5 to 7 months

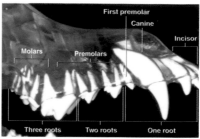

Numbers of roots in maxillary teeth of the dog.

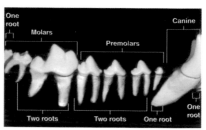

Numbers of roots in mandibular teeth of the dog.

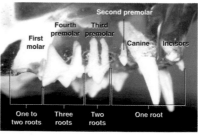

Number of roots in maxillary teeth of the cat.

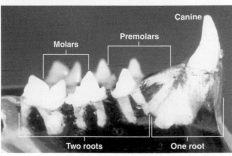

Numbers of roots in mandibular teeth of the cat.

DENTAL TERMINOLOGY[29]

DENTAL ABNORMALITIES

Macrodontia: Oversized crown

Microdontia: Reduced crown

Dilacerated: Distorted (twisted) crown or root

Dens-in-dente: Enamel layer *folds* into itself or tooth

Enamel pearls: Beads of enamel at CEJ, furcation

Fusion tooth: Fusion of two tooth buds during formation

Gemination: Complete tooth duplication but incomplete split

Twinning: Complete tooth duplication and split

Enamel hypocalcification ("hypoplasia"). Enamel pitting and/or discoloration

Hypodontia: Some teeth are missing

Oligodontia: Most teeth are missing

Anodontia: All teeth are missing

Supernumerary: Extra tooth or teeth

DENTAL DIRECTIONAL TERMS

Mesial: Surface of tooth toward the rostral midline

Distal: Surface of tooth away from the rostral midline

Palatal: Surface of tooth toward the palate (maxillary arcade)

Lingual: Surface of tooth toward the tongue (mandibular arcade)

Labial: Surface of tooth toward the lips

Buccal: Surface of tooth toward the cheeks

Facial: Labial and/or buccal surface

Occlusal: Surface of tooth facing a tooth in the opposite jaw

Interproximal: Surface between two teeth

Apical: Toward the apex (root)

Coronal: Toward the crown

Supragingival: Above the gum line

Subgingival: Below the gum line

Mucogingival line (MGL): Junction of the attached gingival and mucosa

Cementoenamel junction (CEJ): Area where the enamel and the cementum meet

DIRECTIONAL TERMS USED IN DENTISTRY[6]

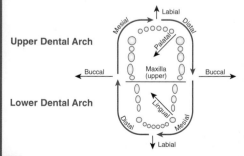

Upper Dental Arch

Lower Dental Arch

Labial · Mesial · Distal · Palatal · Buccal · Maxilla (upper) · Buccal · Distal · Lingual · Mesial · Labial

TOOTH MOBILITY[23]

Grade I: Slight tooth movement
Grade II: Moderate tooth movement of 1 mm
Grade III: Marked tooth movement of more than 1 mm

CLASSIFICATION OF TOOTH FURCATION EXPOSURE[23]

Class I: The furcation can just be detected with a dental probe with very minimal bone involvement.
Class II: The periodontal probe can be placed into the furcation but not all the way through to the other side.
Class III: The periodontal probe can be passed all the way through the furcation to the other side of the tooth.

| Classes of Resorptive Lesions[29] ||
Description	Treatment
Stage 1	
Areas of erosion in the enamel	Use cavity varnish to seal dentinal tubules and harden enamel
Stage 2	
Lesions have penetrated the enamel and dentin	Restore with composite or glass ionomer cavity may varnish; only last 2 years
Stage 3	
Tooth has eroded into the endodontic system	Root canal with restoration; more likely tooth extraction

Continued

Classes of Resorptive Lesions[29]—cont'd

Description	Treatment
Stage 4	
Severe erosion apparent in crown and root structures	Extract tooth
Stage 5	
Crown is totally resorbed	No treatment unless area is inflamed, then extract root

COMMON DENTAL ABBREVIATIONS AND SYMBOLS FOR CHARTING THE MOUTH[29]

X: Extracted

O: Missing

FE: Furcation exposure, or *F1, F2, F3,* grades *1:* furcation detected; *2:* probe passes into furcation; *3:* probe passes through furcation

RE: Root exposure

\: Tooth fracture; also fxo for open fracture, pulp exposed; fxc for closed fracture, no pulp evident

GH: Gingival hyperplasia, charted as *H* followed by number to designate mm (e.g., *H1, H2*)

C: Calculus, charted as *C/H,* heavy; *C/M, moderate; C/S-slight,* an objective decision

CLL, CNL, FRL: Cervical line lesion; cervical neck lesion; feline resorptive lesion *(stage 1 to 4)*

EH: Enamel hypocalcification (hypoplasia)

S: Supernumerary tooth

GR: Gingival recession, charted as *GR* followed by a number to designate mm (e.g., *GR1, GR2*)

M: Mobility, graded 1: slight; 2: moderate; 3: severe with loss of attachment; 4: no longer functional and extraction candidate (e.g., M1, M2, M3)

Gingival scores: *O,* Healthy; *I,* mild gingivitis with slight bleeding upon probing; *II,* moderate gingivitis with edema and erythema and some bleeding; *III,* severe gingivitis with swelling, pustular discharge, pocket formation, bleeding, erythema

CHARTING[34]

NUMBERING TEETH

I. Anatomical system

A. Uppercase letters: permanent teeth

Upper right quadrant	Upper left quadrant
1 if permanent tooth	2 if permanent tooth
5 if deciduous tooth	6 if deciduous tooth
Lower right quadrant	**Lower left quadrant**
4 if permanent tooth	3 if permanent tooth
8 if deciduous tooth	7 if deciduous tooth

B. Lowercase letters: deciduous teeth (primary)

C. Superscript right: upper right teeth

D. Subscript right: lower right tooth

E. Examples

1. I_2: second permanent incisor, lower right

2. ^1c: primary canine, upper left

3. Sp^1: supernumerary first primary premolar, upper right

II. Triadan system
   A. Uses quadrants with three-digit numbers
   B. First number indicates the quadrant in which the tooth is found and the type of tooth
   C. Permanent teeth begin with the numbers 1, 2, 3, and 4
   D. Deciduous (primary) teeth begin with the numbers 5, 6, 7, and 8
   E. The second and third numbers refer to the specific tooth in each quadrant, always beginning from the midline of the mouth
   F. Examples
      1. 103: upper right third permanent incisor
      2. 308: lower left last permanent premolar
   G. Cats are missing teeth 105, 205, 305, 306, 405, 406
   H. Cats

(101-103)	104	(106-108)	109	Upper right
I	C	P	M	
(401-403)	404	407-408	409	Lower right

   I. Dogs

(101-103)	104	(106-108)	109	Upper right
I	C	P	M	
(401-403)	404	407-408	409	Lower right

   J. Rule of 5 and 9
      1. First premolar will always end in a 5
      2. First molar will always end in a 9

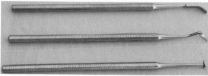

Tartar scrapers are single-ended and used to remove tartar and plaque from the surfaces of teeth.

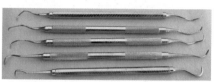

Jacquette tartar scalers are double-ended and used to remove tartar and plaque from the surfaces of teeth.

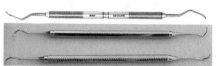

Columbia curets are used to remove tartar from the subgingival surfaces of teeth.

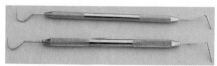

Depth probe and explorer are used to examine teeth for caries, calculi, furcations, and other abnormalities and to explore the depth of the sulci.

■ DENTAL INSTRUMENTS³¹—cont'd ■

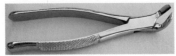

Tooth-splitting and separating forceps are used to split multirooted teeth for removal.

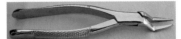

Incisor- and root-extracting forceps grasps the small incisor or the root of a tooth that is to be removed.

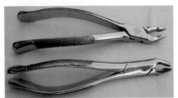

Incisor, canine, and premolar extracting forceps are used to remove incisor, canine, and premolar teeth.

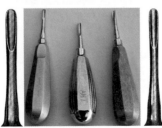

Dental elevators help loosen a tooth from the periodontal ligament before its extraction.

ANESTHESIA MACHINES[18]

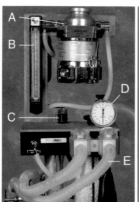
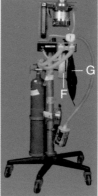

Standard anesthetic machine. Individual components are identified. *A,* Vaporizer; *B,* flowmeter; *C,* oxygen flush valve; *D,* pressure manometer; *E,* circle breathing circuit; *F,* soda lime canister; and *G,* rebreathing bag.

REBREATHING BAG SIZES[4]

$5 \times$ tidal volume = bag size in milliliters (ml). Tidal volume calculated as 10-20 ml/kg of body weight.

Guidelines for Selecting a Bag[33]

500 ml for up to 3 kg
1 L for 4 to 7 kg
2 L for 8 to 15 kg
3 L for 16 to 50 kg
5 L for 51 to 150 kg
30 L for large animals over 150 kg

PERFORMING ANESTHETIC MACHINE CHECK[4]

1. Connect oxygen hose to oxygen source, or turn on local oxygen source.
2. Attach appropriate bag and tubing to be used.
3. Check vaporizer for adequate level of liquid anesthetic.
4. Securely occlude Y-piece with thumb or palm of hand.
5. Completely close pop-off valve.
6. Adjust oxygen flowmeter to 2 L/min.
7. As the rebreathing bag fills with oxygen, the needle gauge on pressure manometer will rise. When the needle reaches 20 cm H_2O, readjust oxygen flow to 200 ml/min.
8. If the system is leak free, the pressure manometer should maintain a reading of 20 cm H_2O for 20 seconds (time with second hand on watch) with the oxygen flowmeter set at 200 ml/min.
9. If the needle gauge declines, there is a leak. Consult the text (or machine manual) for possible locations of leak, and correct.
10. After 20 seconds of a steady needle at 20 cm H_2O, maintain the occlusion on the Y-piece and open the pop-off valve. The rebreathing bag should deflate.
11. Remove thumb from Y-piece.
12. Check scavenging system to ensure connections are intact.
13. Completely open the pop-off valve.

OXYGEN FLOW RATE VALUES[4,33]

Oxygen Flow Rate Quick Look-up Chart for Rebreathing Systems

Guideline Oxygen Flows (L/min)

Weight (kg)	Closed System* (5–10 ml/kg/min, SA)	Semiclosed during Maintenance (20–40 ml/kg/min, SA)	Semiclosed during Induction, Recovery, and Changes (50–100 ml/kg/min, SA)	Semiclosed with Minimal Rebreathing† (200–300 ml/kg/min)
2.5	0.1	0.25	0.25–0.3	0.5–0.8
5	0.1	0.25	0.3–0.5	1–1.5
10	0.1	0.25–0.4	0.5–1	2–3
15	0.1–0.15	0.3–0.6	0.8–1.5	3–4.5
20	0.1–0.2	0.4–0.8	1–2	4–5
25	0.13–0.25	0.5–1	1.3–2.5	5
30	0.15–0.3	0.6–1.2	1.5–3	5
40	0.2–0.4	0.8–1.6	2–4	5

50	0.25–0.5	1–2	2.5–5	5
60	0.3–0.6	1.2–2.4	3–5	5
70	0.35–0.7	1.4–2.8	3.5–5	5
80	0.4–0.8	1.6–3.2	4–5	5
90	0.45–0.9	1.8–3.6	4.5–5	5
100	0.5–1	2–4	5	5
150	0.75–1.5	3–5	5	5

* At flow rates less than 250 ml/min, vaporizer output may not be accurate.

† Minimal rebreathing occurs only when the oxygen flow is greater than or equal to the RMV.

Oxygen Flow Rate Quick Look-up Chart for Non-Rebreathing Systems

Guideline Oxygen Flows (L/min)

Wt. (kg)	Mapleson A (Magill)* Modified Mapleson A (Lack)* Modified Mapleson D (Bain Coaxial)† (0.75–1.0 × RMV)	Modified Mapleson D (Bain Coaxial with No Rebreathing) Mapleson E (Ayre's T-piece) Mapleson F (Norman Mask Elbow and Jackson-Rees) (2–3 × RMV)
1–2.5	0.25–0.5	0.5–1.5
2.5–5	0.5–1	1.5–2.5
5–7	1–1.5	2–3

* Controlled ventilation is not recommended with these systems.
† Flows listed in this column are believed to result in minimal rebreathing with this system during spontaneous ventilation.

ENDOTRACHEAL TUBES[4,33]

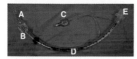

A, Murphy eye; B, cuff; C, cuff indicator; D, body; E, hose connector.

Recommended Endotracheal Tube Sizes[33]	
Species and Body Weight (kg)	Tube Size (Internal Diameter [mm])
Cat	
1	2.5–3
2–4	3.5–4
5 or greater	4.5–5
Dog	
2	5
4	5.5–6
7	6.5–7
10	7.5–8
15	8.5–9
20	9.5–10
25	10.5–11
30	11.5–12
40	13–14

Patient Monitoring Dogs and Cats[4A]		
SaO₂	ETCO₂	Blood Pressure
95%–99%	35–45 mm Hg	Systolic: 90-160 mm Hg Diastolic: 50-90 mm Hg MAP (awake): 85-120 mm Hg MAP (under anesthesia): 70-90 mm Hg

SaO_2, Arterial oxygen saturation, $ETCO_2$, end-tidal carbon dioxide level; *MAP*, mean arterial pressure.

CAPNOGRAPHY

Common Changes in the Capnogram and Associated Causes[33]

Changes	Causes	Capnogram Readout
No waveform	Esophageal intubation Machine malfunction Sensor not properly connected	40 0
Sudden loss of waveform	Apnea Cardiac arrest ET-tube disconnected Accidental extubation Complete ET tube–circuit obstruction Machine malfunction Ventilator malfunction (if using one)	40 0
Gradual decrease in $ETCO_2$	Hypothermia Hyperventilation	40 0

Rapid decrease in ET_{CO_2}	Cardiac arrest Severe blood loss Pulmonary embolism Sudden hypotension	40 0
Gradual increase in ET_{CO_2}	Hypoventilation Malignant hyperthermia Fever Muscle tremors; shivering	40 0
Rapid increase in ET_{CO_2}	Return of spontaneous circulation after successful CPCR	40 0
Increase in baseline CO_2 (usually with gradual increase in E_{CO_2})	Malfunction of expiratory unidirectional valve Saturation of CO_2 absorbent Contamination of sensor with secretions	40 0

Continued

Common Changes in the Capnogram and Associated Causes—cont'd

Changes	Causes	Capnogram Readout
Sudden, temporary increase in ET_{CO_2}	Release of a tourniquet Administration of sodium bicarbonate	
Increased angle of the plateau	Asthma or other obstructive lung disease	
Slow upward stroke	Asthma or other obstructive lung disease Obstructed breathing circuit	
Sloppy upstroke and down-stroke	Leaky cuff Partially kinked endotracheal tube	

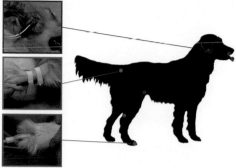

Examples of pulse oximeter probes and locations for placement. Red—transmission probe on the ear flap. Additional red dots show alternate placement locations for this probe (tongue, lip, and flank fold). Green—reflective probe taped to the ventral surface of the tail base. Blue—"C-probe" (a transmission probe) on the toe web. The other blue dot shows an alternate placement location for this probe (the skin fold between the Achilles tendon and the tibia).

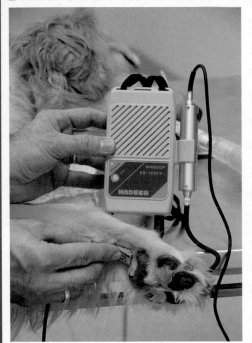

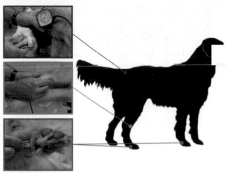

Locations for Doppler probe placement. *Red*, Determination of systolic blood pressure by use of a sphygmomanometer with the cuff placed around the tail base and the probe placed on the ventral surface of the tail distal to the cuff. *Green*, Probe over the dorsomedial surface of the hock. *Blue*, Probe proximal to the metatarsal pad or metacarpal pad

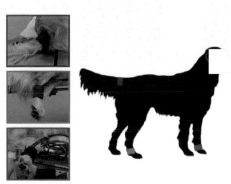

Locations for placement of a blood pressure cuff. Red—base of the tail. Green—metatarsus. Blue—metacarpus.

Electrode Placement for Standard Limb Leads (I, II, III, AVR, AVL, AVF)[7]

RA, white	Right forelimb; clip to skin just proximal to the olecranon (caudal triceps region)
LA, black	Left forelimb; clip to skin just proximal to the olecranon (caudal triceps region)
RI, green	Right hind limb; clip to skin just proximal to the stifle (cranial thigh); ground wire
LL, red	Left hind limb; clip to skin just proximal to the stifle (cranial thigh)

NORMAL CANINE P-QRS-T COMPLEX[10]

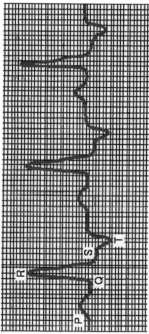

Normal lead II electrocadiographic complex. Atrial depolarization is indicated by the P wave. Following the P wave there is a short delay in the A-V node (P-R segment), after which the ventricles depolarize and produce the QRS complex. This S-T segment and the T wave represent ventricular repolarization.

Common Abnormalities Seen on ECG

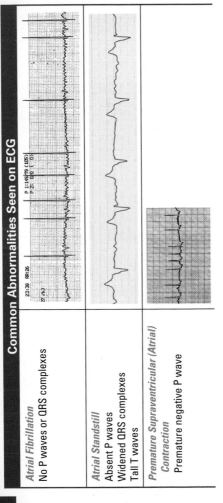

Atrial Fibrillation
No P waves or QRS complexes

Atrial Standstill
Absent P waves
Widened QRS complexes
Tall T waves

Premature Supraventricular (Atrial) Contraction
Premature negative P wave

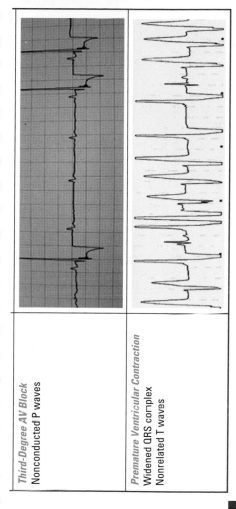

Third-Degree AV Block
Nonconducted P waves

Premature Ventricular Contraction
Widened QRS complex
Nonrelated T waves

American Society of Anesthesiologists Physical Status Classifications[22]

Classification	Risk	Criteria	Representative Conditions
P1	Minimal	Normal, healthy patient	Patients undergoing elective procedures (ovariohysterectomy, castration, or declaw)
P2	Low	Patient with mild systemic disease	Neonatal, geriatric, or obese patients Mild dehydration Skin tumor removal
P3	Moderate	Patient with severe systemic disease	Anemia Moderate dehydration Compensated major organ disease
P4	High	Patient with severe systemic disease that is a constant threat to life	Ruptured bladder Internal hemorrhage Pneumothorax Pyometra

| P5 | Extreme | **Moribund** patient that is not expected to survive without the operation | Severe head trauma
Pulmonary embolus
Gastric dilatation-volvulus
End-stage major organ failure |

Expected Responses of Selected Monitoring Parameters[33]

Stage of Anesthesia	Behavior	Respiration	Cardiovascular Function
I	Disorientation, struggling, fear	Respiratory rate increased; dogs may pant	Heart rate increased
II Excitement stage	Excitement: reflex struggling, vocalization, paddling, chewing	Irregular, may hold breath or hyperventilate	Heart rate often increased

Continued

Expected Responses of Selected Monitoring Parameters[33]—cont'd

Stage of Anesthesia	Behavior	Respiration	Cardiovascular Function
III/Plane 1 Light anesthesia	Unconscious	Regular; rate—high normal	Pulse strong; heart rate high normal
III/Plane 2 Medium (surgical) anesthesia		Regular (may be shallow); rate—moderate	Heart rate moderate
III/Plane 3 Deep anesthesia		Shallow; rate—low or below normal	Heart rate low normal; capillary refill time (CRT) increased; pulse less strong
III/Plane 4		Jerky	Heart rate below normal; prolonged CRT; pale mucous membranes
IV	Moribund	Apnea	Cardiovascular collapse

ASSESSING ANESTHETIC DEPTH[25]

	Indicators of Anesthetic Depth[33]		
Parameter	**Light**	**Medium**	**Deep**
Swallowing	Maybe	No	No
Vaporizer setting	Low (approximately 1 × MAC)	Medium (approximately 1.5 × MAC)	High (approximately 2 × MAC)
Palpebral reflex	Present	Decreased or absent	Absent
Pedal reflex	Present	Absent	Absent
Corneal reflex*	Present	Present	Absent
Pupillary light reflex	Present	May be present	Absent
Spontaneous movement	Maybe	No	No
Muscle tone†	Marked	Moderate	Flaccid
Eyeball position	Usually central	Usually ventromedial	Central

Continued

Indicators of Anesthetic Depth—cont'd

Parameter	Light	Medium	Deep
Pupil size†	Midrange to constricted	Usually midrange	Dilated
Heart rate	Often high or high normal	Often moderate	Often decreased
Respiratory rate	Often high or high normal	Often moderate	Often decreased
Nystagmus (horses)	Fast	Slow	Absent
Salivation, lacrimation	Normal	Decreased	Absent
Response to surgical stimulation	Marked	Moderate	None

* The corneal reflex is not reliable in small animals.

† Strongly influenced by anesthetic protocol and signalment.

Modified from Haskins SC: General guidelines for judging anesthetic depth, *Vet Clin North Am Small Anim Pract* 22:432-434, 1992.

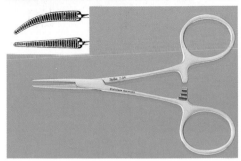

Hartman mosquito forceps

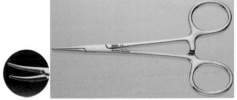

Halstead mosquito forceps

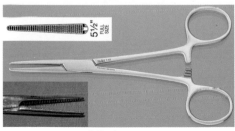

Crile forceps

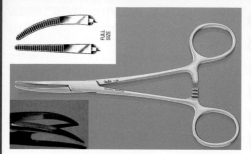

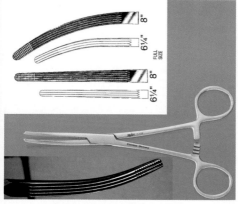

Kelly forceps

Rochester Carmalt forceps

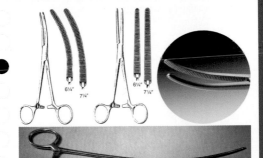

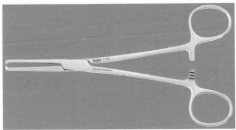

Rochester-Péan forceps

Rochester-Ochsner forceps

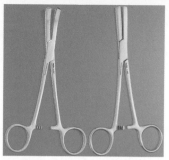

Curved　　**Straight**

Ferguson Angiotribe forceps

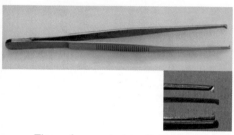

Tissue forceps (rat-tooth forceps)

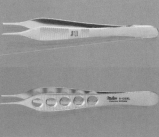

Adson tissue forceps

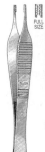
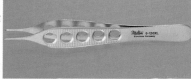

Brown-Adson tissue forceps

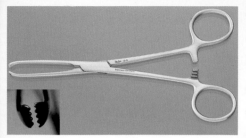

Allis tissue forceps

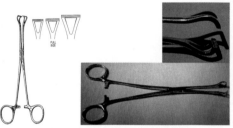

Babcock intestinal forceps

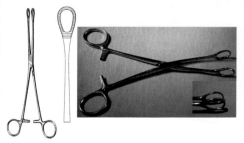

Forester sponge-holding forceps

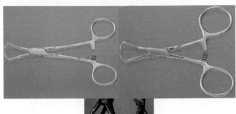

Backhaus towel forceps

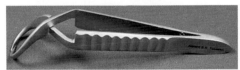

Jones towel forceps

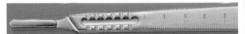

Scalpel handle #4

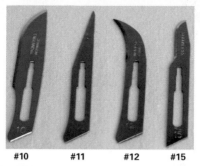

#10   #11   #12   #15

Scalpel blades. #10—A general blade that is used for most procedures in small animals; fits a #3 handle. #11—Used to sever ligaments; fits a #3 handle. #12—Used to lance an abscess; fits a #3 handle. #15—Used for small, precise, or curved incisions.

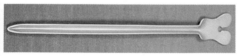

Groove director

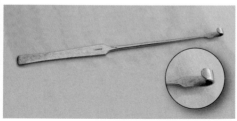

Snook's ovariectomy hook

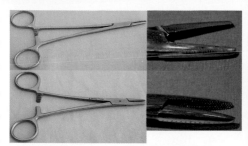

Mayo-Hegar needle holder

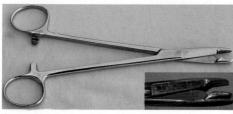

Olson-Hegar needle holder–scissors
combination

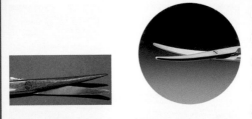

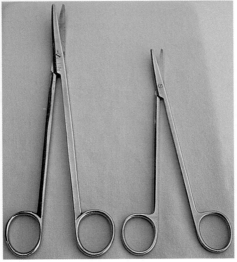

Metzenbaum scissors

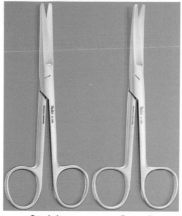

Straight **Curved**

Mayo scissors

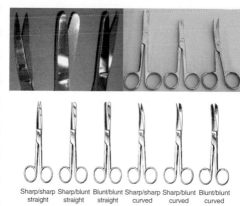

Sharp/sharp Sharp/blunt Blunt/blunt Sharp/sharp Sharp/blunt Blunt/blunt
straight   straight   straight   curved   curved   curved

Operating scissors

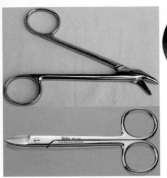

Wire scissors

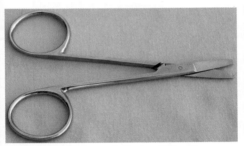

Straight Spencer delicate-stitch scissors

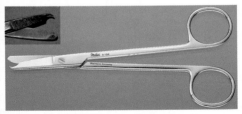

Straight Littauer stitch scissors

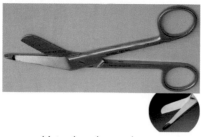

Lister bandage scissors

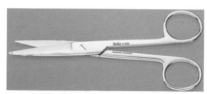

Knowles bandage scissors

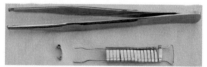

Michel wound clip and applying forceps

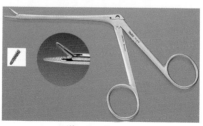

Alligator forceps

189

Suture Material[4]

Generic Name	Brand Name	Absorbability	Multi/Monofilament	Color
Nylon	Ethilon	Nonabsorbable	Mono	Black
Nylon	Dermalon	Nonabsorbable	Mono	Black
Polyester	Surgidac	Nonabsorbable	Multi	Green
Polyester	Ethibond	Nonabsorbable	Multi	Green
Polyglactin 910	Vicryl	Absorbable	Multi	Purple/undyed
Polyglycolic	Dexon-Plus	Absorbable	Multi	Beige
Polypropylene	Surgilene	Nonabsorbable	Mono	Blue
Polypropylene	Prolene	Nonabsorbable	Mono	Blue
Polidioxanone	PDS	Absorbable	Mono	Violet/clear
Silk	Silk	Nonabsorbable	Multi	Black
Chromic gut	Chromic gut	Absorbable	Mono	Beige
Chromic gut	Chromic gut	Absorbable	Mono	Beige
Stainless steel	Surgical steel	Nonabsorbable	Mono	—

Surgical Pack Storage[13]

Wrapper	Shelf Life
Double-wrapped, two-layer muslin	4 weeks
Double-wrapped, two-layer muslin, heat sealed in dust covers after sterilization	6 months
Double-wrapped, two-layer muslin, tape sealed in dust covers after sterilization	2 months
Double-wrapped nonwoven barrier materials (i.e., paper)	6 months
Paper/plastic peel pouches, heat-sealed	1 year
Plastic peel pouches, heat sealed	1 year

Clipping Guidelines for Selected Soft Tissue Surgical Cases

Soft Tissue Procedure/Area	Guidelines
Exploratory laparotomy	Mid-sternum to pubis; laterally to edge of ribs
Gastric, liver, splenic	Mid-sternum to pubis; laterally to edge of ribs
Urinary bladder	Umbilicus to caudal pelvis; laterally to edge of ribs
Kidney	Mid-sternum to pubis; laterally to edge of ribs
Prostate	Umbilicus to caudal pelvis, including prepuce; laterally to edge of ribs
Uterine, ovarian	Xiphoid to pubis; laterally to edge of ribs
Ventral neck	Cranially to mid-mandible; caudally to thoracic inlet; laterally to commissure of lips

Forelimb Area	Guidelines
Digit	Nails to mid-humerus; use towel clamp through nail to suspend limb
Metacarpal	Nails to mid-humerus; use towel clamp through nail to suspend limb
Carpus	Second metacarpal to mid-humerus
Radius, ulna	Mid-metacarpals to shoulder; ventrally to midline; cranially to thoracic inlet; caudally to seventh rib
Elbow	Carpus to dorsal midline; ventrally to ventral midline; cranially to thoracic inlet; caudally to seventh rib
Humerus	Carpus to dorsal midline; ventrally to ventral midline; cranially to base of neck; caudally to seventh rib
Scapula	Mid-radius to 2 clipper-widths past dorsal midline; cranially to base of neck; caudally to tenth rib

Clipping Guidelines for Selected Hindlimb Orthopedic Cases

Hindlimb Area	Guidelines
Digit	Nails to mid-femur; use towel clamp through nail to suspend limb
Metatarsal	Nails to mid-femur; use towel clamp through nail to suspend limb
Tarsus	Second metatarsus to mid-femur
Tibia, fibula	Mid-metatarsals to hip; ventrally to midline; cranially to last rib
Stifle	Tarsus to hip; cranially to last rib; caudally to tuber ischii
Femur	Tarsus to dorsal midline; cranially to last rib; caudally to tuber ischii
Hip	Tarsus to 2 clipper-widths past dorsal midline; cranially to last rib; caudally to tail head
Pelvis	Depends on area of pelvis to have surgery (ilium vs. pubis, vs. ischium); consult surgeon

Clipping Guidelines for Selected Neurologic Surgeries

Vertebrae	Guidelines
Cervical: ventral approach	Midventral mandible to mid-sternum; laterally to halfway between dorsal and ventral midline
Cervical: dorsal approach	Mid-skull to two vertebral spaces caudal to affected space; laterally to half-way between dorsal and ventral midline
Thoracic	Two vertebral spaces cranial and caudal to affected space; laterally to edge of transverse process
Lumbar	Two vertebral spaces cranial and caudal to affected space; laterally to edge of transverse process

Clipping Guidelines for Miscellaneous Surgical Cases

Procedure/Area	Guidelines
Aural	Lateral canthus of eye; dorsal midline on head and neck; ventrally to ventral midline
Ophthalmic: intraocular	Trimming of eyelashes; limited skin clip because of potential irritation
Ophthalmic: extraocular	*Entropion, ectropion:* One clipper-width past lateral canthus, lower lid, and medial canthus *Enucleation:* Midline of muzzle to cranial edge of ear pinna; dorsally to mid-line; ventrally to commissure of lip
Facial	Procedures vary widely among nasal, maxillary, and mandibular; best to consult surgeon
Perineal	Dorsally to tail head; laterally to tuber ischii (bilaterally); ventrally to mid-thigh (caudal aspect)

Signs of Pain	
CARDIOVASCULAR	Elevated heart rate and blood pressure, decreased peripheral circulation, prolonged capillary refill, cool extremities (ears, paws)
RESPIRATORY	Rapid, shallow breaths, panting
DIGESTIVE	Weight loss, poor growth (young), vomiting, inappetence, constipation, diarrhea, salivation
MUSCULOSKELETAL	Unsteady gait, lameness, weakness, tremors, shivering
URINARY	Reluctance to urinate, loss of house training
LABORATORY FINDINGS	Neutrophilia, lymphocytosis, hyperglycemia, polycythemia, elevated cortisol, elevated catecholamines

Postoperative Pain Evaluation

Signs of Pain	Suspected Pain Level	Duration
Head, Ear, Oral, Dental Surgery		
Rubbing; shaking; salivating; reluctance to eat, swallow, or drink; irritability, vocalizing	Moderate to high	Intermittent
Ophthalmologic		
Rubbing, vocalizing, reluctance to move	High	Intermittent to continual
Orthopedic		
Guarding, aggression, abnormal gait, self-mutilation, reluctance to move, dysuria, constipation	Moderate	Intermittent
Abdominal		
Guarding, splinting, abnormal posture, vomiting, inappetence	Mild to moderate	Intermittent
Cardiovascular/Thoracic		
Changes in respiratory rate and pattern, reluctance to move, vocalizing	Moderate to high	Continual
Perirectal		
Licking, biting, scooting, self-mutilation, constipation	Moderate	Intermittent

Pain score 0-10. Choose one descriptor from each category			
Interaction	Awake, willingly interacts, asleep	0	☐
	Awake, responds if encouraged	1	☐
	Awake, reluctant, unwilling	2	☐
Appearance	Asleep, calm	0	☐
	Agitated, vocalizing, looks at injury	1	☐
	Severely agitated, vocalizing, thrashing	2	☐
Posture	Normal, moves easily, asleep	0	☐
	Frequent position changes, guarded gait	1	☐
	Unwilling to lay down, abnormal gait	2	☐
Cardiovascular	HR and/or BP <10% elevated	0	☐
	HR and/or BP 10-20% elevated	1	☐
	HR and/or BP >20% elevated	2	☐
Respiration pattern	Normal	0	☐
	Guarded, mild abdominal	1	☐
	Marked abdominal	2	☐

Numeric pain scale for use in small animal patients. The observer assigns a score for each category. Observations are performed before the animal is physically touched. The overall score is used as a guide as to when to treat or as an assessment of response to treatment.

CATHETER SIZES[12A]

Animal	Urethral Catheter Type	Size (French Units*)
Cat	Flexible vinyl, red rubber, or tom cat catheter (polyethylene)	3.5
Male dog (≤25 lb)	Flexible vinyl, red rubber, or polyethylene	3.5 or 5
Male dog (≥25 lb)	Flexible vinyl, red rubber, or polyethylene	8
Male dog (>75 lb)	Flexible vinyl, red rubber, or polyethylene	10 or 12
Female dog (≤10 lb)	Flexible vinyl, red rubber, or polyethylene	5
Female dog (10-50 lb)	Flexible vinyl, red rubber, or polyethylene	8
Female dog (>50 lb)	Flexible vinyl, red rubber, or polyethylene	10, 12, or 14

*The diameter of urinary catheters is measured on the French (F) scale. One French unit equals approximately 0.33 mm.

■ ROUTINE URINALYSIS PROCEDURE[17] ■

1. Prepare a laboratory sheet with patient information, date, time, and method of urine collection.
2. If sample was refrigerated, make note on the record and allow the sample to warm to room temperature.
3. Properly mix the sample.
4. Record the physical characteristics: color, clarity, volume, and odor of sample by gentle inversion.
5. Calibrate the refractometer with distilled water to 1.000.
6. Determine and record the specific gravity of the sample.
7. Dip a reagent test strip into the urine sample and remove promptly, making sure to tap lightly the edge of the strip on a paper towel to remove excess urine.
8. Read the pad's color at the appropriate time intervals as stated by the manufacturer's directions, and record the results.
9. Properly label a 15-ml conical centrifuge tube.
10. Pour approximately 5 to 10 ml of the urine sample into the centrifuge tube.
11. Centrifuge the sample for 5 to 6 minutes at 1000 to 2000 rpm.
12. Make note of the amount of sediment.
13. Pour off the supernatant, leaving approximately 0.5 to 1 ml in the tube.
14. Resuspend the sediment by gently mixing with a pipette or flicking the tube with the fingers.
15. Transfer a drop of reconstituted sediment to a microscope slide with a transfer pipette, and place a cover slip over it.

16. Alternatively, place 1 drop of Sedi-Stain to 1 drop of urine on a microscope slide, and place a cover slip over it.
17. Subdue the light of the microscope by partially closing the iris diaphragm.
18. Examine the entire specimen under the cover slip with the high power (40×) objective to identify and quantify cells, casts, crystals, and bacteria.
19. To aid in the detection of these elements, the fine adjustment knob should be continuously focused.
20. Record results.

| Gross Examination of Urine[29] ||
Quality	Shows Evidence of
Changes in Color	
Colorless	Dilute urine with low SG; often seen in conjunction with polyuria
Deep amber	Highly concentrated urine (low SG); associated with oliguria
White	Associated with presence of leukocytes
Red to red/brown	Usually indicates presence of RBCs and/or hemoglobin
Changes in Turbidity	
Cloudy	Usually indicates presence of cells (e.g., WBCs, epithelial cells, bacteria)
Milky	Usually indicates presence of fatty material

Continued

Gross Examination of Urine[29]—cont'd	
Quality	**Shows Evidence of**
Changes in Odor	
Sweet	Usually indicates presence of ketones
Pungent	Associated with presence of bacteria
Changes in Volume	
Polyuria	Increase in volume of urine voided in a 24-hour period
Oliguria	Decrease in volume of urine voided in a 24-hour period
Anuria	Absence of urine voiding

■ URINE SEDIMENT EXAMINATION ■

pH Chart for Urine Crystals[17]	
Crystal	**pH**
Ammonium biurate	Slightly acidic, neutral, alkaline
Amorphous phosphate	Neutral, alkaline
Amorphous urates	Acidic, neutral
Bilirubin	Acidic
Calcium carbonate	Neutral, alkaline
Calcium oxalate	Acidic, neutral, alkaline
Cystine	Acidic
Leucine	Acidic
Triple phosphate	Slightly acidic, neutral, alkaline
Tyrosine	Acidic
Uric acid	Acidic

CELLS

Red and White Blood Cells[34,36]

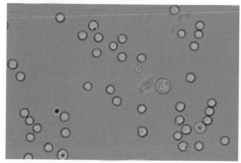

Canine red blood cells and one white blood cell *(right, center)*.

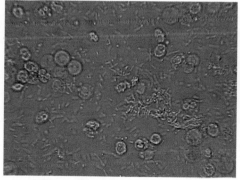

WBCs and bacteria in canine urine.

Epithelial Cells[27]

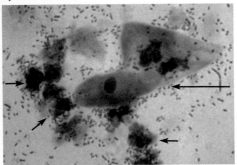

Contaminated urine specimen, free catch, stained. The presence of mature squamous epithelial cells *(long arrow)* suggests the probability of bacterial contamination. Six or seven distorted nuclei, presumably neutrophils, are also observed *(short arrows)*.

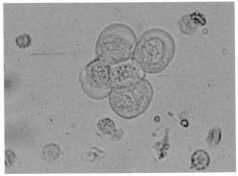

Transitional epithelial cell cluster in canine urine.

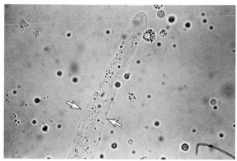

Hyaline cast (×400).

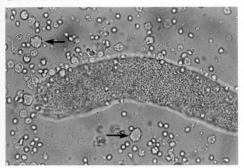

Granular cast, unstained.

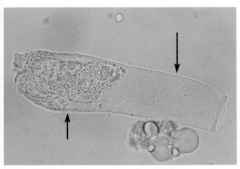

Granular/waxy cast, unstained. Waxy casts develop from granular casts as illustrated by this cast that has granular cast *(short arrow)* and waxy cast *(long arrow)* characteristics.

Cellular Casts[8,27]

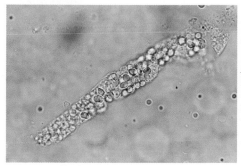

Red cell cast, unstained.

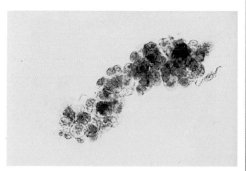

A renal epithelial cast. (Sedi-Stain, original magnification 1120×.)

CRYSTALS

Struvite Crystals[17]

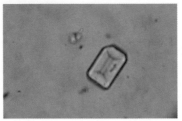

Struvite crystal in canine urine, resembling a coffin lid.

Calcium Oxalate Crystals[22]

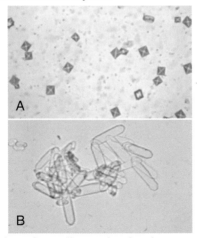

Canine urine sediment showing the two forms of calcium oxalate crystals. **A,** Dihydrate form. **B,** Monohydrate form.

Uric Acid Crystals[26]

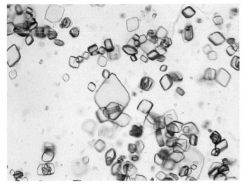

Uric acid crystals are not commonly found in small animals except for Dalmatian dogs.

Amorphous Phosphate Crystals[26]

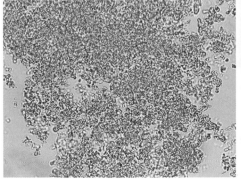

Amorphous phosphate crystals.

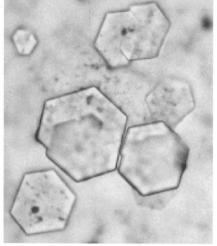

Cystine crystals.

Bilirubin Crystals[27]

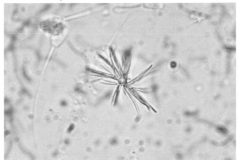

Bilirubin crystals.

Sulfa Crystals[27]

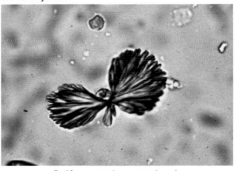

Sulfa crystals, unstained.

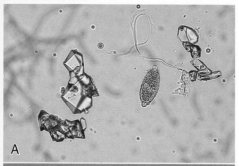

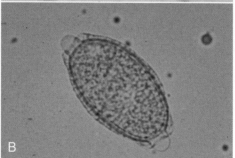

A, *Pearsonema plica* ovum. The ovum of the bladder worm of dogs and cats has slightly tipped bipolar plugs and a granular appearance. (Unstained, HP oil.) **B,** *Pearsonema feliscati,* unstained. Cat. The tilted terminal plugs help identify the ovum. (Unstained; HP oil.)

HEMATOLOGY AND HEMOSTASIS

HEMATOLOGY AND HEMOSTASIS

Anticoagulants[23]		
Color of Top	**Anticoagulant**	**Purpose**
Purple	EDTA	CBC, platelet counts
Red	None	Chemistries
Tiger (red-black)	Separator gel	Chemistries
Green	Heparin	Electrolytes
Turquoise	Citrate	Coagulation assay

Plasma Color and Turbidity[29]

Normal	Clear and colorless to light straw yellow
Icterus	Clear and yellow
Hemolysis	Clear and red
Lipemia	Turbid and white

RBC Indices[29]

Parameter	Equation	Units
MCV	PCV $\times$ 10 RBC count	Femtoliter
MCH	Hb $\times$ 10 RBC count	Picogram
MCHC	Hb $\times$ 100 PCV	Percent

Semiquantitative Evaluation[29]

Number of Cells with Toxic Change	Percentage (%)*
Few	5-10
Moderate	11-30
Many	>30
Observed change	Severity of toxic change
Döhle bodies	Slight
Cytoplasmic basophilia	Slight to marked, depending on intensity
Cytoplasmic vacuolization (foamy cytoplasm)	Moderate to marked, depending on amount
Indistinct nuclear membrane	Marked
Severe cell degeneration	

*If toxic changes occur in less than 5% of neutrophils, they are not reported.

SIZE[17]

Anisocytosis—Variation in the size of the RBCs; seen in splenic or liver disorders; sign of regeneration of anemia

Macrocytosis—RBCs that are larger than normal; represent immature cells; appear as reticulocytes with NMB stain

Microcytosis—RBCs that are smaller than normal; often seen in iron deficiency

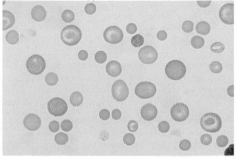

Mixed anisocytosis in a canine blood film. Several target cells are also present.

SHAPE[15,17,35,36]

Normocytic—In K9, appear as biconcave disks; in feline, appear as round cells

Poikilocytosis—Generic term for any abnormally shaped cell; the specific abnormality should be further characterized as appropriate

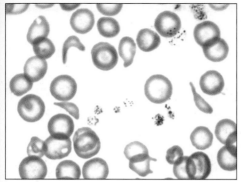

Hypochromic erythrocytes and poikilocytosis.

Schistocytes (schizocyte)—Fragmented RBC; caused by vascular trauma; seen in DIC, neoplasia, etc.

Acanthocytes—Irregular projections from surface of RBC

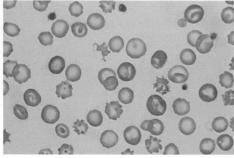

Acanthocytes.

Echinocyte—Scalloped border (regular projections) from surface of RBC

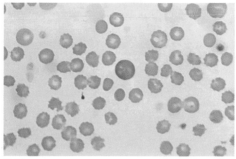

Echinocytes.

Spherocytes—Small dense RBCs with no area of central pallor

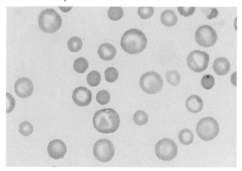

A cluster of four spherocytes, slightly up and left of center, and two spherocytes to the far right of center.

Stomatocyte—RBC with a slitlike center opening; seen in regeneration

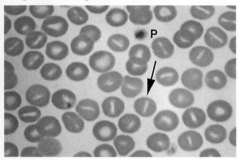

Folded cells and stomatocytes *(arrow)* and a platelet *(P)* on a canine blood film.

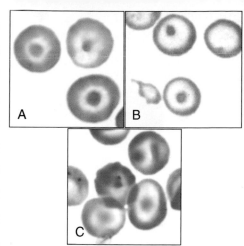

Codocytes in blood from dogs. These erythrocytes exhibit a central density or "bull's-eye" and are often referred to as target cells.

Leptocyte—RBC with an increase in membrane surface relative to cell volume; appear as target cells, codocytes

COLOR

Polychromasia—Cells that exhibit a bluish tint

Hypochromasia—Cells with an increase in the area of central pallor

Hyperchromatophilic—Cells that appear darker than normal; these are often microcytic spherocytes

OTHER ABNORMALITIES[15]

Basophilic stippling—Bluish granular bodies
on the surface of the RBC; seen in regenerative anemia in ruminants; diagnostic for
lead poisoning in small animals

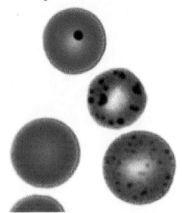

Erythrocytes containing a Howell-Jolly body
(top), diffuse coarse basophilic stippling
(middle), and diffuse fine basophilic stippling
(bottom) in blood from a cat. Wright-Giemsa
stain.

Heinz bodies—Round structures within the RBC representing denatured hemoglobin; small number may be normally present in feline; may be caused by onion toxicity, Tylenol toxicity, etc.

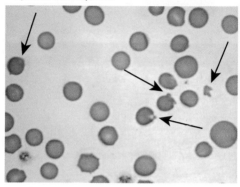

Heinz bodies *(arrows)* are seen on a feline blood film stained with Wright's stain.

Howell-Jolly bodies—Basophilic nuclear remnants in the RBC.

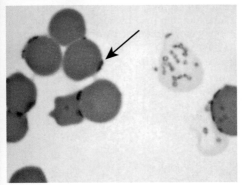

Mycoplasma organisms are seen on the periphery of erythrocytes.

Nucleated RBCs—Seen in regenerative anemias, lead poisoning, extramedullary hematopoiesis, and bone marrow disease

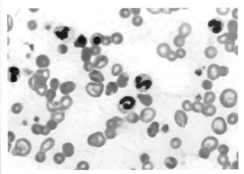

Canine blood film with several polychromatic erythrocytes, two nucleated erythrocytes, and neutrophils.

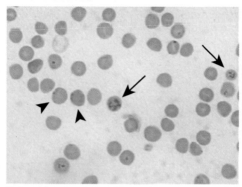

Feline blood smear with both punctuate *(arrowheads)* and aggregate reticulocytes *(long arrows).*

RETICULOCYTE COUNT[23]

$$\frac{\text{\# of reticulocytes}}{1000\ \text{RBCs}} \times 100 = \%\ \text{reticulocytes}$$

$$\begin{array}{l}\text{Corrected} \\ \text{reticulocyte} \\ \text{per unit}\end{array} = \frac{\%\ \text{reticulocytes} \times \text{patient's PCV}}{45\ (\text{dog})\ \text{or}\ 37\ (\text{cat})}$$

Hypersegmentation—Neutrophil nucleus with more than six lobes; associated with a variety of conditions including chronic infection, pernicious anemia, steroid use

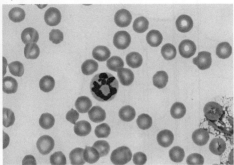

Canine neutrophil with a hypersegmented nucleus.

Karyorrhexis/karyolysis/pyknosis—Describes a nucleus that is condensed, lysed, or damaged; in WBCs in peripheral circulation, these artifacts are caused by the use of inappropriate anticoagulants

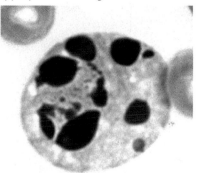

Pyknosis and karyorrhexis of a cell in blood from a dog.

Döhle bodies—Coarse cytoplasmic inclusion representing ribosomal material; common in cats; may be seen with chronic bacterial infection and some viral diseases

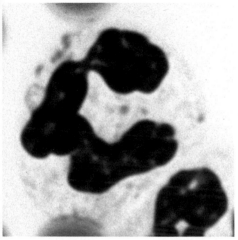

Döhle bodies in the cytoplasm of a neutrophil in blood from a cat.

Vacuolization—One of several toxic changes seen in both lymphocytes and neutrophils; associated with septicemia; also produced as an artifact if sample is held in anticoagulant for extended time; found in normal monocytes

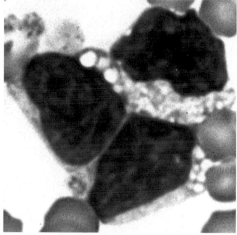

Lymphocytes with cytoplasmic vacuoles in the blood of a cat.

Toxic granulation—Appearance of numerous large granules that range in color from dark purple-red or black; seen in most infectious diseases

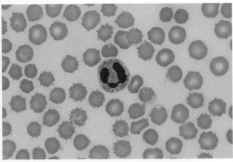

Toxic granulation in a canine neutrophil. The cell also shows cytoplasmic basophilia and foaminess.

Band cell—Immature WBCs (usually neutrophils) with nonsegmented nucleus; nuclear sides are usually parallel

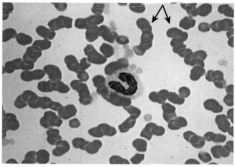

A neutrophilic band cell is present along with marked rouleaux *(arrows)* in a blood film.

Reactive lymphocytes—Cells with dark-blue cytoplasm and darker nucleus; seen in chronic infection

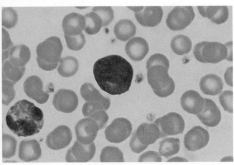

A large, reactive lymphocyte in a cat with abundant basophilic cytoplasm and prominent, pale perinuclear golgi region. (Wright's stain, original magnification 330×.)

Atypical lymphocytes—Refers to a variety of changes in lymphocytes including eosinophilic cytoplasm and changes in nuclear texture

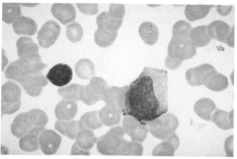

Atypical lymphocytes. The cell on the left is a normal small lymphocyte with a compact nucleus filling the entire cytoplasm. The atypical lymphocyte on the right has abundant cytoplasm and a large nucleus with fine chromatin.

Basket cell—Common term used to describe degenerative WBCs that have ruptured; also referred to as *smudge cells;* may be an artifact if blood is held too long before making the smear; also associated with leukemia

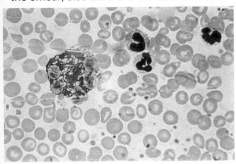

A smudge cell and several neutrophils in a canine blood film.

CORRECTED WBC COUNT[17]

$$\text{Corrected WBC count} = \text{Observed WBC count} \times \frac{\%\ \text{NRBCs}}{100\ \text{WBCs}}$$

PLATELET ESTIMATE[17]

$$\frac{\text{Thrombocytes}}{100\ \text{leukocytes}} \times \frac{\text{WBC count}}{\mu l} = \frac{\text{thrombocytes}}{\mu l}$$

MATERIALS
- Bleeding time device
- Gauze strip
- Filter paper or gauze sponges
- Timing device

PROCEDURE[11]
1. Place animal in lateral recumbency.
2. Expose mucosal surface of upper lip. Position a gauze strip around the maxilla to fold up the upper lip. Tie the strip gently, just tight enough to partially block venous return.
3. The incision site should be void of surface vessels and slightly inclined so that blood shed from the incision can flow freely toward the mouth. Place bleeding time device flush against mucosal surface, applying as little pressure as possible; press tab to release scalpels.
4. Let stab incisions bleed freely and undisturbed until bleeding stops. Excessive blood should be blotted as often as necessary to avoid blood flow into the patient's mouth. Place either filter paper or gauze sponge approximately 3 to 4 mm below the incision, taking care not to disturb the incision site and any clot that may be forming.

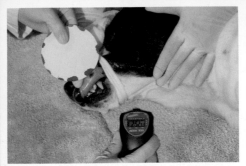

Determination of the buccal mucosal bleeding time in a dog.

5. The endpoint is recorded when the edge of the filter paper or sponge does not soak up free-flowing blood. The bleeding time is the mean bleeding time for the two incisions.

CLINICAL CHEMISTRY AND IMMUNOLOGY

BLOOD CHEMISTRY TESTS[34]

LIVER FUNCTION TESTS
- AST (aspartate aminotransferase)
- ALT (alanine aminotransferase)
- AP (alkaline phosphatase)
- Total serum bilirubin
- Direct-conjugated bilirubin
- Bile acids
- Glucose
- Cholesterol
- Urine bilirubin
- Urine urobilinogen
- Total serum protein

- Serum albumin
- Electrophoresis: protein fractionation
- Plasma fibrinogen
- Hematology

KIDNEY FUNCTION TESTS
- Serum creatinine
- Blood urea nitrogen
- Urine concentration and water deprivation tests
- Endogenous creatinine clearance tests
- Serum electrolytes and minerals: sodium, potassium, calcium, phosphorus, magnesium, chloride
- Hematology

PANCREATIC FUNCTION TESTS

Endocrine Function
- Serum glucose
- Urinalysis; urine glucose
- Glucose tolerance tests

Exocrine Function
- Serum amylase
- Serum lipase
- Trypsinlike immunoreactivity assay

TESTS FOR MUSCLE DISEASE
- Creatine kinase
- AST
- LDH

DIGESTIVE TRACT TESTS
- Serum amylase
- Serum lipase
- Fecal trypsin
- Examine feces for parasites, fat, starch, muscle fibers
- Plasma turbidity test
- Glucose tolerance test

Immunology Tests[17A]

Product Name	Type of Test
Allergies	
Allercept	ELISA
Bile Acids Test	
SNAP Bile Acids	ELISA
Blood Typing Test	
RapidVet-H	Agglutination test
RapidVet-H IC	Immunochromato-graphic assay
Borreliosis, Heartworm, and Ehrlichia canis	
SNAP 3 Dx Test	ELISA
Borreliosis, Heartworm, Ehrlichia, and Anaplasma	
SNAP 3DX Test	ELISA
Brucellosis	
Herdchek: Anti BLV abortus test	ELISA
D-Tec CB	Agglutination test
Canine Pancreas-Specific Lipase	
SNAP cPL	ELISA
Feline Infectious Peritonitis	
Virachek/CV	ELISA
Cushing Syndrome, Addison Disease	
SNAP Cortisol	ELISA
Feline Leukemia Virus	
Assure/FeLV	ELISA
SNAP FeLV antigen test kit	ELISA
Virachek/FeLV	ELISA
WITNESS FeLV	RIM

Continued

Immunology Tests[17A]—cont'd

Product Name	Type of Test
Feline Leukemia Virus and Immunodeficiency Virus	
SNAP Combo	ELISA
Feline Heartworm, Feline Leukemia Virus and Immunodeficiency Virus	
SNAP Feline Triple	ELISA
Feline Pancreas-Specific Lipase	
SNAP fPL	ELISA
Giardia	
SNAP *Giardia*	ELISA
Heartworm Infection	
Petchek	ELISA
Dirochek	ELISA
Heska Solo Step FH & CH	Lateral flow immunoassay
SNAP Heartworm RT Test	ELISA
Witness HW	ELISA
Hypothyroidism and Hyperthyroidism	
SNAP Total T_4, SNAP T_4	ELISA
Mycoplasma Species	
Mycoplasma plate antigens	Plate agglutination test
Ovulation Timing	
ICG Status-LH	Immunochromatographic assay
Parvovirus Infection	
Assure Parvo	ELISA
SNAP canine parvovirus antigen test kit	ELISA

Continued

Immunology Tests[17A]—cont'd

Product Name	Type of Test
Pregnancy, Canine	
Witness Relaxin	RIM
Progesterone	
Ovuchek Premate	ELISA
Rheumatoid Arthritis	
Synbiotics CRF (canine rheumatoid factor)	Latex agglutination
Tuberculin PPD	Intradermal test

■ FECAL FLOTATION PROCEDURE[17] ■

- Materials
- Flotation solution
- Shell vial or test tube and test tube rack
- Waxed paper cups
- Cheesecloth cut into 6- × 6-inch squares
- Wooden tongue depressor
- Microscope slides and cover slips

PROCEDURE

1. Take approximately 2 g ($^1/_2$ tsp) of feces and place it in the cup. Add 20 ml of flotation solution. With a tongue depressor, mix the feces and flotation solution until no large fecal pieces remain.
2. Wrap cheesecloth around the lip of the cup while bending the cup to form a spout. Pour the mixture through the cheesecloth into a vial. Fill the vial so that a meniscus is formed. If the cup does not have enough fluid, fill the vial with as much mixture as available and then fill the remainder with flotation solution.
3. Gently place a cover slip on top of the vial.

Continued

FECAL FLOTATION PROCEDURE[17]—cont'd

4. Allow the unit to remain undisturbed for 10 to 20 minutes (sugar solution requires a longer waiting time than sodium nitrate). If the preparation is not allowed to sit this long, some eggs will not have time to float to the surface. If allowed to sit for more than an hour, some eggs may become waterlogged and sink or the eggs may become distorted.
5. Carefully remove the cover slip by picking it straight up and placing it on a microscope slide with the wet side adjacent to the slide.
6. Examine the area of the slide under the cover slip with the 10× objective. Record any parasitic material found in the sample.

CENTRIFUGAL FLOTATION PROCEDURE[17]

MATERIALS

- Same as for standard flotation, but omit the vials
- 15-ml centrifuge tube
- Microscope slides and cover slips

PROCEDURE

1. Prepare the fecal mixture as described in the standard flotation procedure.
2. Strain the mixture through cheesecloth into the 15-ml centrifuge tube. Fill the tube to the top. (If using a fixed-rotor centrifuge, the tube should be filled halfway and a cover slip should not be used.) Apply a cover slip to the top of the tube. Always balance the centrifuge with a 15-ml tube filled with flotation solution and a cover slip placed on top. Be sure all tubes are marked with patient identification information after centrifugation.

CENTRIFUGAL FLOTATION PROCEDURE[17]—cont'd

4. Remove the cover slip or use a wire loop or glass rod to remove the top part of fluid in the tube and place on a microscope slide. Microscopically examine the sample with the 10× objective.

FECAL SEDIMENTATION PROCEDURE[17]

MATERIALS
- Waxed paper cups
- Cheesecloth cut in 6- × 6-inch squares
- Wooden tongue depressors
- Centrifuge and 15-ml tubes
- Pasteur pipettes with bulbs
- Microscope slides and cover slips

PROCEDURE
1. Mix approximately 2 g of feces with tap water in a waxed paper cup. Strain the mixture through cheesecloth into a centrifuge tube, filling the tube half full.
2. Balance the centrifuge with tubes filled with equal amounts of water. Centrifuge for 3 to 5 minutes at 1300 to 1500 rpm. If a centrifuge is unavailable, allow the tube to sit undisturbed for 20 to 30 minutes.
3. Slowly pour the liquid off the top without disturbing the sediment layer (including the fine, silty material) on the bottom.
4. Using a pipette, transfer a small amount of the fine sediment to a microscope slide. Apply a coverslip to the drop of sediment and examine microscopically. Lugol's iodine may be mixed with the drop of sediment before a coverslip is applied; this facilitates identification of protozoal cysts or trophozoites.

MATERIALS

- 15-ml centrifuge tube
- Centrifuge
- 2% formalin (2 ml of 40% formalin diluted with 98 ml of distilled water)
- Methylene blue stain (diluted 1:1000 with distilled water)
- Pasteur pipettes and bulbs

PROCEDURE

1. Mix 1 ml of blood with 9 ml of 2% formalin in a centrifuge tube.
2. Centrifuge the tube at 1300 to 1500 rpm for 5 minutes.
3. Pour off the liquid supernatant, leaving the sediment at the bottom of the tube.
4. Add 2 to 3 drops of stain to the sediment. Using a pipette, mix the sediment with the stain.
5. Place a drop of this mixture onto a glass slide. Apply a cover slip and examine microscopically.

COMPARISON OF *DIROFILARIA* AND *ACANTHOCHEILONEMA* (*DIPETALONEMA*)[29]

Characteristic	*Dirofilaria immitis*	*Dipetalonema reconditum*
Body shape	Usually straight	Usually curved
Body width	5-7.5 μ	4.5-5.5 μ
Body length	295-325 μ	250-288 μ
Cranial end	Tapered	Blunt
Caudal end	Straight	Curved or hooked
Numbers	Numerous	Sparse
Movement	Undulating	Progressive

Dirofilaria immitis[16]

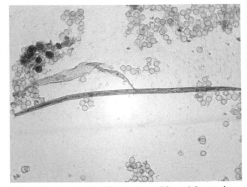

Microfilaria of *Dirofilaria immitis* subjected to modified Knott's test. Note the tapering anterior end and straight tail.

Dirofilaria immitis[16]

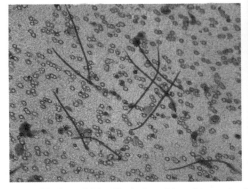

Microfilariae of *Dirofilaria immitis* subjected to commercially available filter technique.

Ancylostoma caninum[16]

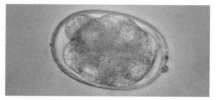

Eggs of *Ancylostoma* spp. and *Uncinaria* spp. are oval or ellipsoidal, thin walled, and contain an 8- to 16-cell morula when passed in feces.

Trichuris vulpis[16]

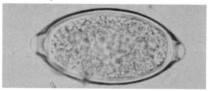

Characteristic egg with a thick, yellow-brown, symmetric shell with polar plugs at both ends.

Toxocara canis[16]

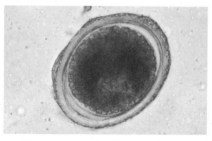

Egg of *Toxocara canis* with unembryonated, spherical form with deeply pigmented center and rough, pitted outer shell.

Toxascaris leonina[16]

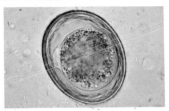

Eggs of *Toxascaris leonina* have a smooth outer shell and hyaline or "ground glass" central portion.

Dipylidium caninum[16]

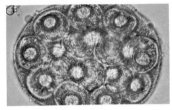

Egg packets, each containing 20 to 30 hexacanth embryos.

Taenia egg[16]

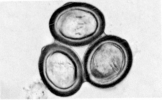

Typical taeniid egg with striated shell and six inner hooks. Egg is characteristic for tapeworms of genera *Taenia, Multiceps,* and *Echinococcus.*

Giardia species trophozoite[16]

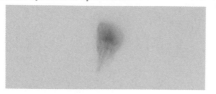

Giardia species trophozoite

Giardia lamblia cyst[3]

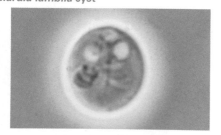

Giardia lamblia cyst

Eimeria magna oocysts[3A]

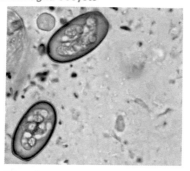

Eimeria oocysts, sporulated (×425)

Isospora felis oocysts[3]

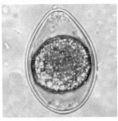
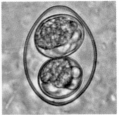

Isospora felis unsporulated *(left)* and sporulated oocyst *(right)* (×1074)

■ COMMON EXTERNAL PARASITES ■

Trichodectes canis[3]

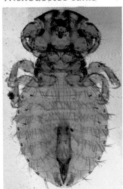
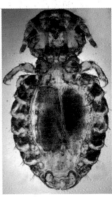

Trichodectes canis

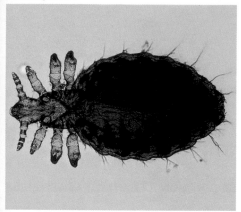

Sucking louse *Linognathus setosus* of dogs

Adult *Sarcoptes scabei* mite[16]

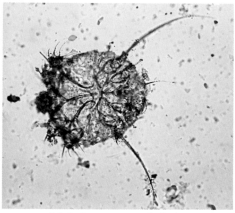

Adult *Sarcoptes scabei* mite

Sarcoptes scabei eggs[16]

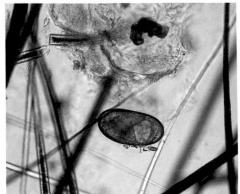

Oval eggs of *Sarcoptes scabei*; note emergence of six-legged larval mite.

Otodectes cynotis[16]

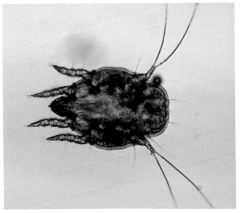

Adult male ear mite, *Otodectes cynotis*

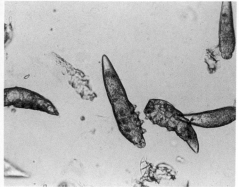

Demodex criceti, a hamster mite, is distinguishable from *Demodex aurati* by its blunt body shape.

Egg of *Demodex canis*[16]

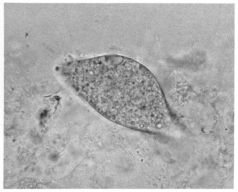

Egg of *Demodex canis* is either spindle shaped or tapered at each end.

Commonly Used Culture Media[23A]

Purpose and Inoculation	Reaction and Interpretations
Blood Agar Plate (Trypticase Soy Agar with 5% Sheep Blood)	
Primary isolation medium for colony isolation.	Observe growth rates, colony morphologic characteristics, hemolysis.
MacConkey Agar	
Primary isolation and differential plating medium for selection and recovery of *Enterobacteriaceae* and related gram-negative bacteria.	Growth is usually gram negative. Pink-to-red colonies (with increased redness of the medium) are lactose fermenters. Colorless colonies (often with a slight change of the medium-to-yellow) are nonlactose fermenters.
Selenite Broth or Tetrathionate Broth	
Enrichment broth for the selective enhancement of growth by *Salmonella*.	Subculture to MacConkey agar and Hektoen enteric agar for isolation of *Salmonella*.

Triple Sugar Iron (TSI) Agar Slant

Differential medium for detection of carbohydrate fermentation and production of hydrogen sulfide. Inoculate by stabbing the butt and streaking the slant. Incubate with a loose cap.	Yellow color change indicates acidification caused by carbohydrate fermentation. Results are recorded as slant/butt: A, acid (yellow); K, alkaline (red); or NC, no change.

Motility Media*

For determining whether an organism is motile or nonmotile. Inoculate by stabbing the center of the tube with an inoculating needle.	Motile organisms migrate from the stab line, flaring out to cause turbidity in the medium. Nonmotile organisms grow only along the stab line; the surrounding medium remains clear.

Indole Test Media*

Used for detecting the ability of bacteria to produce indole from tryptophan metabolism. Incubate 24-48 hr, then add Kovac's reagent to detect indole.	Development of a red color at the interface of the reagent and the broth within seconds after adding the reagent indicates a positive test result.

*Combination media that provide for several tests in the same tube, such as SIM (sulfide-indole-motility), MIO (motility indole ornithine), or MIL (motility indole lysine), can be purchased.

Sample Collection Guidelines[17A]

Acceptable Specimen	Transport Device	Comments
Central Nervous System		
Spinal fluid	Blood culture medium	Hold, ship at RT
Blood		
Whole, unclotted blood Minimum of 3 ml	Blood culture medium	Hold, ship at RT Submit ≤3 samples per 24 hr collected during febrile spike
Eye		
Conjunctival swab Corneal scrapings Ocular fluid	Amies or semisolid reducing medium Syringe	Hold, ship at RT Inoculate plated media directly with corneal scrapings if fungal keratitis suspected
Bone and Joints		
Joint aspirate Bone marrow aspirate, bone	Blood culture medium Sterile tube	Hold, ship at RT

Urinary Tract		
Urine by cystocentesis Catheterized urine Midstream urine	Sterile tube	Hold, ship under refrigeration
Upper Respiratory Tract		
Nasopharyngeal swab Sinus washings Biopsy specimen	Semisolid reducing medium Sterile tube	Ship refrigerated except washings, biopsies (RT)
Lower Respiratory Tract		
Transtracheal wash Lung aspirate or biopsy	Sterile tube Semisolid reducing medium	Hold, ship at RT
Gastrointestinal Tract		
Feces Rectal swab	Sterile cup or bag Cary-Blair or semisolid reducing medium	Feces: hold, ship at RT; refrigerate *Campylobacter, Brachyspira* suspects

Continued

Sample Collection Guidelines[17A]—cont'd

Acceptable Specimen	Transport Device	Comments
Skin		
Aspirate or swab, if superficial	Sterile syringe semisolid-reducing medium	Anaerobe suspects not refrigerated
Deep swab of draining tract	Sterile tube with saline	
Tissue biopsy	Paper envelope	
Scabs, hairs, scrapings		
Milk		
Remove milk from teat cistern; collect 5-10 ml aseptically	Sterile tube	Freeze
Necropsy Tissue		
Lesions, including adjacent, normal tissue	Whirl-Pak bags	Individual containers to prevent cross-contamination; ship refrigerated
Minimum of 1 cm³ to maximum of 35 cm³	Screw-cap jars	

Necropsy Tissue—cont'd		
Include one serosal or capsular surface intact		
Reproductive Tract		
Prostatic fluid, raw semen	Sterile tube	
Uterus	Biopsy or swab	Guarded swabbing for uterine cultures; hold, ship at RT
Vagina		
Abortion	Fetal lung, liver, kidney, stomach contents, placenta in separate Whirl-Pak bags or screw-capped containers	Ship refrigerated

RT, Room temperature.

1. Collect specimen.
2. Direct Gram stain of specimen.
3. Inoculate culture media.
4. Incubate 18 to 24 hours.
5. Check for growth.
   a. If negative (no growth):
      (1) Reincubate.
      (2) Recheck.
      (3) If no growth, report as "no growth."
   b. If positive (colonies on media):
      (1) Select representative colonies.
      (2) Direct Gram stain.
      (3) Continue with identification procedures (e.g., additional media, biochemical testing).

■ QUADRANT STREAK PROCEDURE[17] ■

1. Use a sterile bacteriologic loop to remove a small amount of the bacterial colony from the culture plate or a loopful from a broth culture.
2. Optional: Divide a plate into four quadrants by marking the bottom of the Petri dish with a black marker.
3. Hold the loop horizontally against the surface of the agar to avoid digging into the agar when streaking the inoculum.
4. Lightly streak the inoculating loop over one quarter (quadrant A) of the plate using a back-and-forth motion; keep each streak separate.
5. Pass the loop through a flame and allow it to cool.
6. Place the inoculating loop on the edge of quadrant A, and extend the streaks into quadrant B using a back-and-forth motion.

7. Pass the loop through a flame and allow it to cool.
8. Place the inoculating loop on the edge of quadrant B, and extend the streaks into quadrant C using a back-and-forth motion.
9. Pass the loop through a flame and allow it to cool.
10. Place the inoculating loop on the edge of quadrant C, and extend the streaks into quadrant D using a back-and-forth motion.

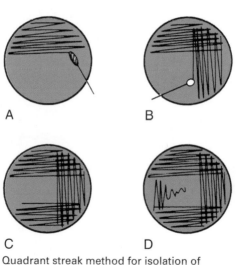

A

B

C

D

Quadrant streak method for isolation of bacteria.

Common Bacterial Pathogens[17A]

	Blood Agar	MacConkey Agar	Other Characteristics
Gram-Positive			
Staphylococcus	Smooth, glistening, white-to-yellow pigmented colonies	No growth	Catalase-positive glucose fermenter; double-zone hemolysis usually indicates coagulase positive; coagulase activity is a useful differential test
Streptococcus	Small, glistening colonies; hemolysis	No growth except some enterococci	Catalase negative, usually identified by type of hemolysis; beta-hemolytic strains more likely to be pathogens; others are often part of flora; *Streptococcus agalactiae* camp positive
Corynebacterium renale	Small, smooth, glistening colonies (24 hr); become opaque and dry later	No growth	Catalase positive; urease positive

Listeria monocytogenes		
Small, hemolytic, glistening colonies	No growth	Catalase positive; motile at room temperature
Nocardia		
Slow-growing, small, dry, granular, white-to-orange colonies	No growth	Partially acid fast; colonies tenaciously adhere to media
Clostridium		
Variable, round, Ill-defined, irregular colonies; usually hemolytic	No growth	Obligate anaerobes
Bacillus		
Variable, large, rough, dry, or mucoid colonies	No growth	Usually hemolytic; large rods with endospores
Gram-Negative		
Escherichia coli		
Large, gray, smooth mucoid colonies; hemolysis variable	Hot pink-to-red colonies; red cloudiness in media	Hemolysis frequently associated with virulence

Continued

Common Bacterial Pathogens[17A]—cont'd

	Blood Agar	MacConkey Agar	Other Characteristics
Gram-Negative—cont'd			
Klebsiella pneumoniae	Large, mucoid, sticky whitish colonies; not hemolytic	Large, mucoid, pink colonies	Nonmotile; require biochemical tests to differentiate from *Enterobacter*
Proteus	Frequently swarming without distinct colonies	Colorless; limited swarming	
Other Enterics	Gray to white, smooth, mucoid colonies	Colorless colonies	Biochemical tests for identification; serotyping indicated for *Salmonella*
Pseudomonas	Irregular, spreading, grayish colonies: variable hemolysis; may show a metallic sheen	Colorless, irregular colonies	Oxidase positive; fruity odor; may produce yellow-to-greenish soluble pigment in clear media

Bordetella bronchiseptica		
Very small, circular dew-drop colonies; variable hemolysis	Small, colorless colonies	May require 48 hr for distinct colonies; oxidase positive; rapid urease positive; citrate positive
Brucella canis		
Very small, circular, pinpoint colonies after 48-72 hr; not hemolytic	No growth	Oxidase positive; catalase positive; urease positive
Moraxella		
Round, translucent, grayish-white colonies; variable hemolysis	No growth	Oxidase and catalase positive; often nonreactive in routine biochemical tests; colonies may pit media
Antinobacillus		
Round, translucent colonies; variable hemolysis	Variable growth; colorless colonies	Glucose fermenter, nonmotile; urease positive; sticky colonies
Pasteurella multocida		
Gray, mucoid, round to coalescing colonies; no hemolysis	No growth	Glucose fermenter in TSI; weak oxidase and indole positive

cAMP, Cyclic adenosine monophosphate; *TSI*, triple sugar iron (agar).

BACTERIAL COLONY CHARACTERISTICS[17]

Form

  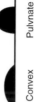

Punctiform   Circular   Filamentosus   Irregular   Rhizod   Spindle (lens)

Elevation

Flat   Raised   Convex   Pulvnate   Umbonate

Margin

Entire (even)   Undulate (wavy)   Filamentous   Lobate (lobes)   Erose (serrated)   Curled

Bacterial colonies may be described on the basis of their form, elevation, and margins.

Characteristics of Yeasts[17]

Genus	Pseudohyphae	True Hyphae	Blastoconidia	Arthroconidia	Urease	Growth at 25°C with Cycloheximide	Growth at 37°C on Potato Dextrose Agar
Candida	+	+	+	–	–	Var	+
Geotrichum	–	+	–	+	–	–	–
Malassezia	–	–	–	–	+	+	+
Trichosporon	–	–	+	+	+	+	+

Var, Variable.

Microsporum canis[30]

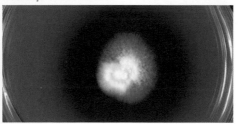

Microsporum canis on dermatophyte test medium

Microsporum canis[30]

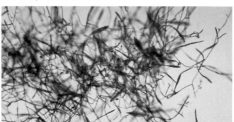

Microsporum canis macroconidia

Trichophyton mentagrophytes[30]

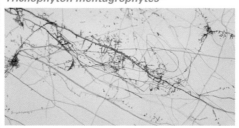

Trichophyton mentagrophytes macroconidia

SKIN SCRAPE PROCEDURE[17]

1. For biopsy specimens, use a scalpel blade to expose a fresh edge of the tissue.
2. Blot the sample until it is nearly dry.
3. Hold the blade at a 90-degree angle, and scrape across the tissue.
4. Spread the sample onto a clean slide.
   a. Use a motion similar to spreading peanut butter.
   b. If the sample appears thick on the slide, make a compression smear from it.
5. Air dry the slide before staining by gently waving it in the air.

FINE NEEDLE BIOPSY TECHNIQUES

ASPIRATION PROCEDURE[17]

1. Stabilize mass.
2. Insert needle.
3. Retract plunger to create negative pressure.
4. Redirect the needle several times.
   a. Do not exit the mass.
   b. Maintain negative pressure.
5. Remove needle from mass.
6. Remove syringe from needle.
7. Fill syringe with air.
8. Reattach needle.
9. Gently force sample from needle onto clean slide.
10. Air dry the slide before staining by gently waving it in the air.

NONASPIRATE PROCEDURE[17]

1. Stabilize mass.
2. Insert needle (may have a syringe barrel attached without the plunger).
3. Redirect the needle several times.

Continued

    a. Do not exit the mass.

    b. Maintain negative pressure.

4. Remove needle from mass and remove syringe barrel (if used) from needle.

5. Fill syringe with air.

6. Reattach needle.

7. Gently force sample from needle onto clean slide.

8. Air dry the slide before staining by gently waving it in the air.

COMPRESSION SMEAR PREPARATION[17]

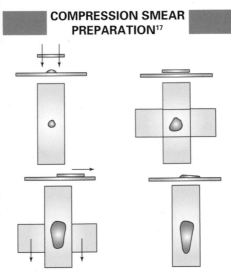

A portion of the aspirate is expelled onto a glass microscope slide. Another slide is placed over the sample, spreading the sample. The slides are smoothly slipped apart, which usually produces well-spread smears.

TRACHEAL WASH[9]

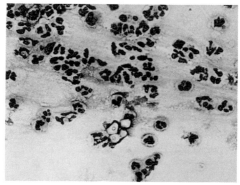

High numbers of neutrophils, an alveolar macrophage, and a cluster of four granules of cornstarch from glove powder in a tracheal wash sample.

APPEARANCE OF EFFUSIONS[17]

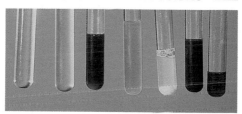

Gross appearance of various effusion *(left to right)*: clear and colorless; yellow and slightly turbid; hemolyzed and slightly turbid; orange and turbid; sedimented fluid; bloody; and turbid, brown, and slightly turbid.

Characteristics of Fluid Samples[17]

	Transudate	Exudate	Normal	Modified Transudate
Origin				
	Noninflammatory hypoalbuminemia Vascular stasis Neoplasia	Inflammatory Infection Necrosis		Feline infectious peritonitis Chylous effusion Lymphatic fluid
Amount of Fluid				
	Large	Variable	Small	Variable
Color				
	Clear, colorless, or red tinged	Turbid, white, slightly yellow	Clear, colorless	Variable, usually clear
Protein				
	<3.0 g/dl	>3.0 g/dl	<2.5 g/dl	2.5-7.5 g/dl

TNCC			
<1500/ml	>5000/ml	<3000/ml	1000-7000/ml
Cell Types			
Mixture of monocytes, macrophages, lymphocytes, and mesothelial cells* (normal and/or reactive)	Inflammatory: neutrophils, macrophages, lymphocytes,* and eosinophils*	Same as transudate	Lymphocytes, nondegenerate neutrophils, mesothelial cells, macrophages, and neoplastic cells

*Variable numbers.

Nuclear Criteria of Malignancy[9A]

Nuclear Criteria and Description	Schematic Representation
Macrokaryosis	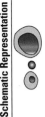
Increased nuclear size. Cells with nuclei larger than 10 mcg in diameter suggest malignancy.	
Increased Nucleus: Cytoplasm Ratio (N:C)	
Normal nonlymphoid cells usually have an N:C of 1:3 to 1:8; depending on the tissue. Ratios ≥1:2 suggest malignancy.	
Anisokaryosis	
Variation in nuclear size. This is especially important if the nuclei of multi-nucleated cells vary in size.	
Multinucleation	
Multiple nucleation in a cell. This is especially important if the nuclei vary in size.	
Increased Mitotic Figures	Normal Abnormal
Mitosis is rare in normal tissue.	

276

Abnormal Mitosis

Chromosomes are improperly aligned.

Coarse Chromatin Pattern

The chromatin pattern is coarser than normal. It may appear ropy or cordlike.

Nuclear Molding

Nuclei are deformed by other nuclei within the same cell or adjacent cells.

Macronucleoli

Nucleoli are increased in size. Nucleoli ≥5 μ strongly suggest malignancy. For reference, RBCs are 5 to 6 μ in cats and 7 to 8 μ in dogs.

Angular Nucleoli

Nucleoli are fusiform or have other angular shapes; instead of their normal round to slightly oval shape.

Anisonucleoliosis

Nucleolar shape or size varies. This is especially important if the variation is within the same nucleus.

Characteristics of Tumor Types[17]

Tumor Type	Cell Size	Cell Shape	Cellularity	Clumps or Clusters
Epithelial	Large	Round to caudate	Usually high	Common
Mesenchymal	Small to medium	Spindle to stellate	Usually low	Uncommon
Discrete round cell	Small to medium	Round	Usually high (except histiocytoma)	Uncommon

COMMON CELL TYPES IN CYTOLOGY SAMPLES

SUPPURATIVE INFLAMMATION[26]

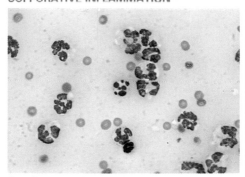

Suppurative inflammation as evidenced by the large number of neutrophils. Note the presence of karyorrhexis in the center cell.

PYOGRANULOMATOUS INFLAMMATION[9]

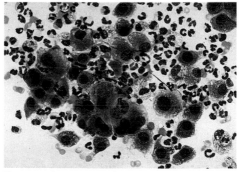

Pyogranulomatous inflammation. Macrophages represent more than 15% of the cells present.

SEPTIC INFLAMMATION[9]

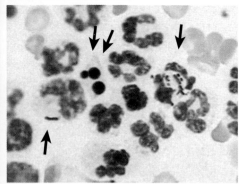

Septic inflammation. Degenerated neutrophils with phagocytized bacterial rods *(arrows)*. A pyknotic cell *(double arrows)* is also present.

CARCINOMA[9]

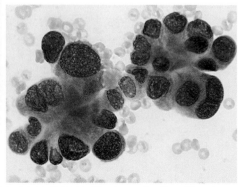

Lung carcinoma. Clusters of cells with aniso-karyosis, binucleation, and high and variable nucleus/cytoplasm ratios.

SARCOMA[9]

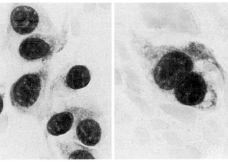

Sarcoma. Aspirate from a malignant spindle cell tumor with cells showing anisokaryosis; anisonucleiosis; and large, prominent, and occasionally angular nucleoli.

PLASMA CELLS[9]

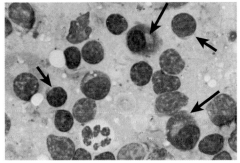

Several plasma cells are evident in this sample *(long arrows)* from a hyperplastic lymph node. Small lymphocytes are also present *(short arrows)*.

MESOTHELIAL CELLS[9]

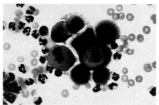

A cluster of reactive mesothelial cells. Note the mitotic figure.

PYOGRANULOMATOUS LYMPHADENITIS[26]

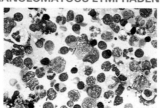

Pyogranulomatous lymphadenitis. Numerous macrophages and neutrophils are evident along with a mixture of lymphocyte types.

EAR SWABS

MALESSIZIA ORGANISMS[9]

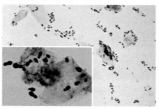

Sample from an ear swab containing *Malassezia* organisms.

CELL TYPES FOUND IN LYMPH NODE ASPIRATES[17]

Lymphocytes, small—Similar in appearance to the small lymphocyte seen on a peripheral blood film. Slightly larger than an RBC. Scanty cytoplasm, dense nucleus.

Lymphocytes, intermediate—Nucleus approximately twice as large as an RBC; abundant cytoplasm.

Lymphoblasts—Two to four times as large as the RBC. Usually contains a nucleolus. Diffuse nuclear chromatin.

Plasma cells—Eccentrically located nucleus, trailing basophilic cytoplasm, perinuclear clear zone. Vacuoles and/or Russell bodies may be present.

Plasmablasts—Similar to lymphoblasts with more abundant, basophilic cytoplasm. May contain vacuoles.

Neutrophils—May appear similar to neutrophil in peripheral blood or show degenerative changes.

Macrophages—Large phagocytic cell. May contain phagocytized debris and microorganisms. Abundant cytoplasm.

Mast cells—Round cells that are usually slightly larger than lymphoblasts. Distinctive purple-staining granules may not stain adequately with Diff-Quik.

Carcinoma cells—Epithelial tissue origin. Usually found in clusters; pleomorphic.

Sarcoma cells—Connective tissue origin. Usually occur singly with spindle-shaped cytoplasm.

Histiocytes—Large, pleomorphic, single or multinuclear; nuclei are round to oval.

PARABASAL CELLS[9]

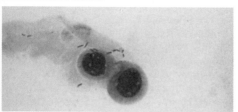

Parabasal vaginal epithelial cells from a dog.

INTERMEDIATE VAGINAL EPITHELIAL CELLS[9]

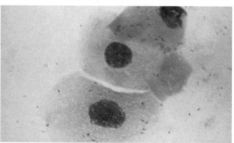

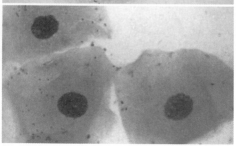

Small and large intermediate vaginal epithelial cells from a dog.

SQUAMOUS CELL[9]

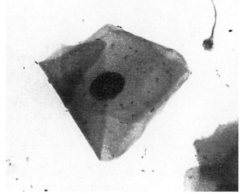

Superficial epithelial cell with a slightly pyknotic nucleus and folded angular cytoplasm.

CORNIFIED CELLS[9]

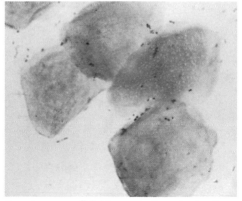

Anuclear superficial (cornified) vaginal epithelial cells from a dog.

PROESTRUS[9]

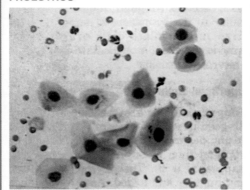

Vaginal smear from a dog in proestrus. Intermediate epithelial cells predominate. Red blood cells and a few neutrophils are also present.

DIESTRUS[9]

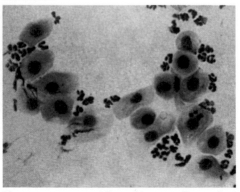

Numerous neutrophils and intermediate cells from a vaginal smear of a dog in diestrus.

Normal Blood Gas Values[2]				
Sample	pH	Pco_2 (mm Hg)	HCO_3 (mm Hg)	Po_2 (mm Hg)
Dog venous	7.32-7.40	33-50	18-26	
Dog arterial	7.36-7.44	36-44	18-26	85-100
Cat venous	7.28-7.41	33-45	18-23	
Cat arterial	7.36-7.44	28-32	17-22	85-100

*In-house normal values should be established if the machine does not come with a published reference range.

Normal Daily Urine Production for Dogs and Cats[17A]

Species	Daily Urine Output (ml/kg)
Dogs	20-40
Cats	20-40

Normal Heart Rate and Blood Pressure in Dogs and Cats[12]

Normal Heart Rate (Beats/Min)	Normal Blood Pressure (mm Hg)		
	Systolic	Diastolic	Mean
Dogs (Large)			
60-100	100-160	60-90	80-120
Dogs (Medium)			
80-120	100-160	60-90	80-120
Dogs (Small)			
90-140	100-160	60-90	80-120
Cats			
140-200	100-160	60-90	80-120

Normal Physiologic Data in Adult Dogs and Cats[29]

	Heart Rate (Beats/Min)	Respiratory Rate (Breaths/Min)	Rectal Temperature
Dogs	70-160	8-20	37.5°-39.0° C
Cats	150-210	8-30	38°-39° C

Hematology Reference Range Values[12]

Test	Adult Canine	Adult Feline	Units
Red blood cell (total)	5.32-7.75	6.68-11.8	× 10^6 cells/μl
Hemoglobin (Hgb)	13.5-19-5	11.0-15.8	g/dl
Hematocrit (Hct)	39.4-56.2	33.6-50.2	%
Mean corpuscular volume (MCV)	65.7-75.7	42.6-55.5	fL
Mean corpuscular hemoglobin (MCH)	22.57-27.0	13.4-18.6	pg
Mean corpuscular hemoglobin concentration (MCHC)	34.3-36.0	31.3-33.5	g/dl
Platelet count	194-419	198-405	× 10^3 cells/μl
Mean platelet volume (MPV)	8.8-14.3	11.3-21.3	fL
White blood cell (total)	4.36-14.8	4.79-12.52	× 10^3 cells/μl
Segmented neutrophils (segs)	3.4-9.8	1.6-15.6	× 10^3 cells/μl
Nonsegmented neutrophils (bands or nonsegs)	0-0.01	0-0.01	× 10^3 cells/μl
Lymphocytes (lymphs)	0.8-3.5	1.0-7.4	× 10^3 cells/μl
Monocytes (monos)	0.2-1.1	0-0.7	× 10^3 cells/μl
Eosinophils (eos)	0-1.9	0.1-2.3	× 10^3 cells/μl
Basophils (basos)	0	0	× 10^3 cells/μl

Normal Chemistry[12]

Test	Adult Canine	Adult Feline	Units
Glucose	73-116	63-150	mg/dl
Blood urea nitrogen (BUN)	8-27	15-35	mg/dl
Creatinine (Cr)	0.5-1.6	0.5-2.3	mg/dl
Phosphorus (P)	2.0-6.7	2.7-7.6	mg/dl
Calcium (Ca)	9.2-11.6	7.5-11.5	mg/dl
Ionized calcium (iCa)	1.15-1.39	—	mg/dl
Total protein (TP)	5.5-7.2	5.4-8.9	g/dl
Albumin (Alb)	2.8-4.0	3.0-4.2	g/dl
Globulin (Glob)	2.0-4.1	2.8-5.3	g/dl
Cholesterol (Ch)	138-317	42-265	mg/dl
Bilirubin (total)	0-0.2	0.1-0.5	mg/dl
Alkaline phosphatase (SAP or Alk Phos)	15-146	0-96	IU/L

Alanine aminotransferase (ALT)	16-73	5-134	IU/L
Gamma glutamyltransferase (GGT)	3-8	0-10	IU/L
Creatine kinase (CK; formerly CPK)	48-380	72-481	IU/L
Potassium (K)	147-154	147-165	mEq/L
Sodium (Na)	3.9-5.2	3.3-5.7	mEq/L
A:G ratio	0.6-2.0	0.4-1.5	—
Na:K ratio	27.4-38.4	30-43	—
Chloride (Cl)	104-117	113-122	mEq/L
Bicarbonate (venous)	20-29	22-24	mEq/L
Anion gap	16.5-28.6	15-32	—
Osmolality (calculated)	292-310	290-320	mOsm/kg
Amylase	347-1104	489-2100	IU/L
Lipase	22-216	0-222	mg/dl
Triglyceride (TG)	19-133	24-206	

Normal Urinalysis Values[12]

Test	Canine	Feline
Specific gravity (SpGr)	Variable	Variable
Color	Pale-to-dark yellow	Pale-to-dark yellow
pH	5.0-8.5	5.0-8.5
Protein	Negative to +1	Negative to +1
Glucose	Negative	Negative
Ketones	Negative	Negative
Bilirubin	Negative to trace	Negative
Blood	Negative	Negative
Microscopic		
Red blood cell (RBC) count	<5 RBCs/hpf	<5 RBCs/hpf
White blood cell (WBC) count	<3 WBCs/hpf	<3WBCs/hpf
Epithelial cells	Negative	Negative
Casts	Negative	Negative
Bacteria	Negative	Negative
Special: urine protein: creatinine	<0.3	<0.6

Hemostasis Reference Range Values[12]

Tests	Canine	Feline
Platelet count	166-600 $\times 10^3$/µl	230-680 $\times 10^3$/µl
Prothrombin time (PT)	5.1-7.9 sec	8.4-10.8 sec
Activated partial thrombo-plastin time (APTT)	8.6-12.9 sec	13.7-30.2 sec
Fibrin degrada-tion products (FDP)	<10 µg/ml	<10 µg/ml
Fibrinogen	100-245 mg/dl	110-370 mg/dl
Activated clotting time (ACT)	60-110 sec	50-75 sec

Summary of the Lengths of the Estrous Cycle and Gestation Periods in Dogs and Cats[23]

Puberty	Estrous Cycle Length	Estrus Duration	Ovulation	Optimal Breeding (Fresh/Frozen)	Gestation
Canine					
6 months	No true cycle (estrus is 2 times/yr)	9 days	2-4 days after onset of cytologic estrus	Days 3 and 5 or 4 and 6 after LH peak/day 5 or 6 after LH peak	57 days from first day of cytologic diestrus or 63 days from ovulation or 65 days from LH peak
Feline					
6-12 months	Seasonally polyestrous and depends on whether ovulation occurs	8 days	Induced ovulators after coitus	After third day of estrus and >2 hr apart for at least three breedings	65 days

SOURCES

An "A" in the reference citation indicates that material was adapted from the source cited.

1. Battaglia A: *Small animal emergency and critical care,* ed 2, St Louis, 2007, Elsevier.
2. Bill R: *Clinical pharmacology and therapeutics for the veterinary technician,* ed 3, St Louis, 2006, Elsevier.
3. Bowman D: *Georgis' parasitology for veterinarians,* ed 9, St Louis, 2009, Saunders.
4. Busch: *Small animal surgical nursing: skills and concepts,* St Louis, 2006, Elsevier.
5. Colville T, Bassert JM: *Clinical anatomy and physiology for veterinary technicians,* ed 2, St Louis, 2008, Elsevier.
6. Colville T, Bassert JM: *Clinical anatomy and physiology laboratory manual for veterinary technicians,* St Louis, 2009, Elsevier.
7. Coté E: *Clinical vet advisor: dogs and cats,* St Louis, 2007, Saunders.
8. Cowell RL, Rick L: *Diagnostic cytology and hematology of the dog and cat,* ed 3, St Louis, 2008, Mosby.
9. Cowell RL, Tyler RD, Meinkoth JH: *Diagnostic cytology and hematology of the dog and cat,* ed 2, St Louis, 1999, Mosby.
10. Edwards NJ: *ECG manual for the veterinary technician,* St Louis, 1993, Saunders.
11. Feldman EC, Ettinger SJ: *Textbook of veterinary internal medicine,* ed 7, St Louis, 2010, Saunders.
12. Ford F, Mazzaferro E: *Kirk and Bistner's handbook of veterinary procedures and emergency treatment,* ed 8, St Louis, 2006, Saunders.
13. Fossum T: *Small animal surgery,* ed 3, St Louis, 2007, Mosby.
14. Han C, Hurd C: *Practical diagnostic imaging for the veterinary technician,* ed 3, St Louis, 2003, Mosby.
15. Harvey JW: *Veterinary hematology,* St Louis, 2012, Saunders.
16. Hendrix CM, Robinson E: *Diagnostic parasitology for veterinary technicians,* ed 3, St Louis, 2006, Mosby.
17. Hendrix CM, Sirois M: *Laboratory procedures for veterinary technicians,* ed 5, St Louis, 2007, Mosby.
18. Holmstrom S: *Veterinary dentistry for the technician and office staff,* St Louis, 2000, Saunders.
19. Kumar V: *Robbins basic pathology,* ed 8, St Louis, 2008, Saunders.
20. Maggs DJ, Miller PE, Ofri R: *Slatter's fundamentals of veterinary ophthalmology,* ed 4, St Louis, 2008, Saunders.

21. McBride DF: *Learning veterinary terminology,* ed 2, St Louis, 2002, Mosby.
22. McCurnin DM, Bassert JM: *McCurnin's clinical textbook for veterinary technicians,* ed 7, St Louis, 2010, Saunders.
23. McCurnin DM, Bassert JM: *Clinical textbook for veterinary technicians,* ed 6, St Louis, 2006, Saunders.
24. McCurnin DM, Bassert JM: *Clinical textbook for veterinary technicians,* ed 5, St Louis, 2002, Saunders.
25. McKelvey D, Hollingsworth KW: *Veterinary anesthesia and analgesia,* ed 3, St Louis, 2003, Mosby.
26. Raskin RE, Myer DJ: *Atlas of canine and feline cytology,* St Louis, 2001, Saunders.
27. Raskin RE, Meyer DJ: *Canine and feline cytology,* ed 2, St Louis, 2010, Saunders.
28. Sheldon CC, Sonsthagen T, Topel J: *Animal restraint for veterinary professionals,* St Louis, 2006, Mosby.
29. Sirois M: *Principles and practice of veterinary technology,* ed 2, St Louis, 2004, Mosby.
30. Songer JG, Post KW: *Veterinary microbiology: bacterial and fungal agents of animal disease,* St Louis, 2005, Saunders.
31. Sonsthagen T: *Veterinary instruments and equipment: a pocket guide,* St Louis, 2006, Mosby.
32. Taylor SM: *Small animal clinical techniques,* St Louis, 2010, Saunders.
33. Thomas JA, Lerche P: *Anesthesia and analgesia for veterinary technicians,* ed 4, St Louis, 2011, Mosby.
34. Tighe M, Brown M: *Mosby's comprehensive review for veterinary technicians,* ed 3, St Louis, 2008, Mosby.
35. Willard MD, Tvedten H: *Small animal clinical diagnosis by laboratory methods,* ed 5, St Louis, 2012, Saunders.
36. Sirois M: *Principles and practice of veterinary technology,* ed 3, St Louis, 2011, Mosby.
37. Chew DJ, DiBartola SP, Schenck PA: *Canine and feline nephrology and urology,* ed 2, St Louis, 2011, Saunders.
38. Tear M: *Small animal surgical nursing,* ed 2, St Louis, Mosby, 2012.
39. Case LP: *Canine and feline nutrition,* ed 3, St Louis, 2011, Mosby.
40. McCurnin DM, Poffenbarger EM: *Small animal physical diagnosis and clinical procedures,* St Louis, 1991, WB Saunders.